SKIN CARE
for Teens

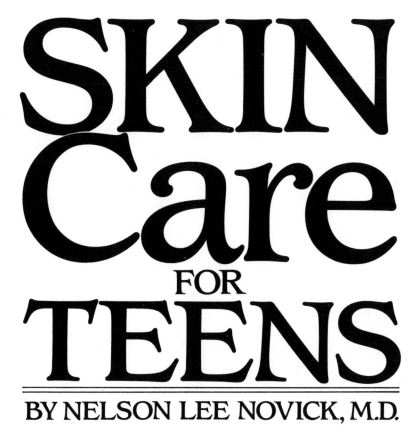

SKIN Care

FOR
TEENS

BY NELSON LEE NOVICK, M.D.

Franklin Watts
New York/London/Toronto/Sydney/1988

Illustrations by Anne Canevari Green

Library of Congress Cataloging-in-Publication Data

Novick, Nelson Lee.
Skin care for teens.

Includes index.
Summary: A dermatologist discusses acne treatment,
make-up, rashes and infections, and skin, nail, and
foot care.
1. Skin—Care and hygiene—Juvenile literature.
2. Youth—Health and hygiene—Juvenile literature.
[1. Skin—Care and hygiene. 2. Grooming] I. Title.
RL87.N69   1988   646.7'26   87-27909
ISBN 0-531-10521-0

Contents

SKIN CARE
for Teens

Preface

Your skin is the largest organ of your body. It weighs about 7 pounds (3.15 kg) and stretches some 20 square feet (1.8 sq m). It serves many vital functions, including protection and temperature regulation. In addition, your skin acts like a mirror of your mind and body, reflecting the way you feel emotionally or physically. The relationship between your skin and your health and feelings is so strong that even our everyday speech contains such common expressions as "white as a sheet," "flushed with excitement," and "blushing like a bride." Some of you have probably noticed that when you're anxious, sick for several days, or haven't gotten enough sleep, your skin may become pale or sallow and your eyes may develop dark circles under them. On the other hand, when you are feeling well and are well rested, your skin usually shows it. When you feel happy or excited, for example, after winning a sports match or getting a 100 on an exam, your skin may appear to glow.

Your skin has to last you a lifetime. What you do or don't do for it now can make a big difference in how you look and feel, not only now but for the rest of your life. Your skin, hair, and nails must be routinely and properly cared for in order to remain healthy and attractive. It's a rare individual indeed who can do little or nothing for his or her skin and be lucky enough to continue having it.

Knowing the facts about skin, hair, and nail care is essential for looking and feeling your best. Much of what you already know about skin care and skin-care products probably comes from your friends or relatives, or from television, newspapers, and popular magazines. Unfortunately, in many cases, the information contained in TV and radio commercials, product advertisements, or on product labels is frequently incorrect, incomplete, or misleading. In some cases, it may even be intentionally fraudulent. Unless you know some basic information about skin, hair, and nails, and the products and conditions that affect them, you can needlessly waste your time and your money. Even worse, your appearance and health can suffer.

This book begins by providing factual medical and scientific information about your skin. You'll learn its structure and function, as well as how to keep your skin more attractive and healthy. In Chapter 2, you'll learn how to read and understand a cosmetic ingredient label. You'll learn to make sense out of a long list of confusing-sounding ingredients. You'll also learn how to choose beauty aids and grooming products more sensibly. In short, you'll learn what to look for and what to watch out for when buying products for your skin.

Chapters 3, 4, and 5 discuss in nontechnical language the causes, prevention, and treatment of a variety of common skin conditions. These include oily skin, acne, eczema, psoriasis, boils, warts, and ringworm, to name just a few. Wherever appropriate, an effort is made to dispel popular misconceptions about any of these conditions.

Chapter 6 covers frequent hair and scalp problems and hair-care products; Chapter 7, nails and the safe use of nail-care products; and Chapter 8, your feet and how best to care for them. In Chapter 9, special problems, such as excessive sweating, and treatment of special areas of your body with unique problems, are discussed.

Finally, since cosmetic surgery has grown so popular, no book on skin would be complete without a discussion of the more common surgical ways to change the way you look. Chapter 10 describes procedures for improving noses, fixing ears, changing chins, removing scars, and eliminating certain skin discolorations.

Throughout the book, you will find many different medications referred to either by their brand or generic names. The specific products or ingredients mentioned are those with which I have had considerable personal experience in my practice and which I have found to be consistently helpful; this should not, however, be misunderstood to be an endorsement of any product(s). The specific products mentioned are by no means the only ones available for treating any particular condition. However, where some products or therapies have been found to be worthless, it is clearly stated.

This book is intended to make you knowledgeable about the proper care and treatment of your skin, hair, and nails. The advice offered in this book is of a general nature and is not intended to be relied upon as a substitute for the advice of, or consultation with, your doctor. Naturally, if you have any specific questions about any product, skin condition, or treatment, you should ask your dermatologist.

1

Keeping Skin Healthy

NORMAL SKIN STRUCTURES AND FUNCTIONS

The skin is a complex organ that serves many functions. Most importantly, it protects the inside of your body from the outside environment and helps to regulate your body temperature. Figure 1.1 is a cross section of normal skin, showing its various layers.

Skin is divided into three main layers: a cellular upper layer, called the *epidermis;* a fibrous middle layer, called the *dermis;* and a fatty lower layer, called the *subcutis.* The top layer of the epidermis is covered by a sheet of ready-to-be-shed dead skin cells called the *horny layer.* The horny layer is the major physical barrier to the environment. It protects against invasion by germs and to a limited extent protects against the rays of the sun.

The lowest level of the epidermis is composed of two types of cells: *basal cells* and *melanocytes.* Basal cells divide and reproduce, continually giving birth to new cells. These newly formed cells in turn mature and rise to the surface of the epidermis to replenish the continuously shed horny layer.

—13—

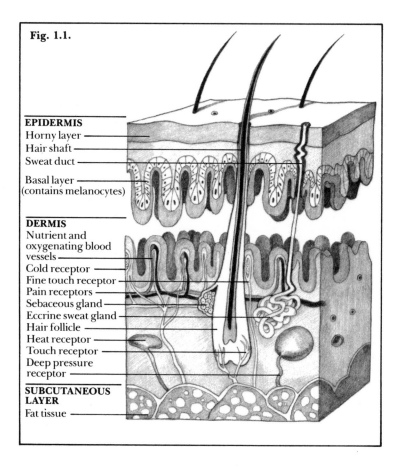

Fig. 1.1.

EPIDERMIS
Horny layer
Hair shaft
Sweat duct
Basal layer
(contains melanocytes)

DERMIS
Nutrient and
oxygenating blood
vessels
Cold receptor
Fine touch receptor
Pain receptors
Sebaceous gland
Eccrine sweat gland
Hair follicle
Heat receptor
Touch receptor
Deep pressure
receptor
SUBCUTANEOUS
LAYER
Fat tissue

Human Skin

Melanocytes are cells that produce the skin pigment *melanin,* which is responsible for giving a brownish color to skin. Melanin is capable of absorbing the sun's ultraviolet rays and thus protects the skin from damaging ultraviolet radiation. Racial differences in skin color are largely inherited differences in the amount and distribution of melanin.

The dermis is the supporting layer of the skin. It is composed of cells and fibers. The dermis also contains many small blood vessels that provide nutrition for the skin. Oxygen and nutrients for your skin are *not* supplied through the surface of the skin but by the blood vessels within the dermis.

Certain product manufacturers, particularly those producing moisturizing lotions, "rejuvenating" lotions, and antiaging or antiwrinkling lotions, try to sell you on the idea that your skin can "drink" or "eat up" the ingredients in their products. Despite these misleading or exaggerated advertising claims, your skin cannot soak up most substances applied to it. The molecules in these too-good-to-be-true "magic" elixirs and potions are simply too large to pass through the skin into the dermis. They merely coat the skin and nothing more. Moisturizers are discussed in greater detail later in this chapter.

Sebaceous glands (oil glands), hair roots, and sweat glands lie within the subcutis, the fat layer of your skin. (Depending upon the location on the body, these same structures may also be found in the dermis.) *Sebum*, which is the name for the oily fluid produced by the sebaceous glands, coats your hair and skin, giving it a sheen, keeping it smooth and supple, and locking in moisture. Sweat glands help to regulate body temperature through the evaporation of perspiration. The fat content of the subcutis itself serves as an energy source and also as a cushion to protect underlying tissues from injury.

PROTECTING AND PRESERVING YOUR SKIN

It's a fact of life that for better or worse you will have to live with your skin for the rest of your life. What you do to your skin today can have dramatic effects on what it does to you or for you later. In general, following measures to keep your skin healthy requires that you know something about three fundamental areas of skin care: sun protection, cleansing, and moisturizing (when needed).

Sun Protection

WARNING: THE SURGEON GENERAL HAS DETERMINED THAT SUNTANNING IS DANGEROUS TO YOUR HEALTH. SUNTANNING MAY LEAD TO THE DEVELOPMENT OF PREMATURE AGING, SAGGING, WRINKLING, AND DISCOLORATION OF YOUR SKIN, AND THE DEVELOPMENT OF SKIN CANCERS.

Unfortunately, you won't find this warning on billboards advertising suntanning products or in advertisements for "getaway" travel packages to sun-drenched Florida or the Caribbean. However, overwhelming medical and scientific evidence points to the sun as Public Enemy #1 of your skin.

Since the 1920s, when suntans became fashionable, a golden brown tan has been considered a sign of good health. Like the great outdoors and mountain air, it was assumed that the sun, being part of nature, could only be good for you. The sun was even believed to possess curative powers. As an example, not long ago, mothers frequently sent their children outdoors to bask in the sun to "dry up a cold."

Unquestionably, the sun has some beneficial effects. Vitamin D is important for bone development and growth, and sunlight is capable of stimulating vitamin D production in your skin. In addition, it can't be denied that many people find basking in the warm sun a psychologically refreshing experience. Finally, a deep tan can mask acne blemishes or other discolorations or irregularities of the skin.

Unhappily, if you are an avid "sun worshiper" and love to spend all your free time in the sun, you will probably be quite upset to learn that the risks of sun exposure far outweigh any of its benefits. These include severe wrinkling, leathery texture, the development of numerous reddish "broken" blood vessels, reddish scaly precancers, skin cancers, and discolorations. Other effects include freckling, the occasional development of whiteheads, lip cracking and damage, and permanent loss of skin color in certain areas of your skin. Sun exposure has also been linked to the development of a potentially fatal form of skin cancer, *malignant melanoma*, which can attack people even in their teens, twenties, and thirties.

Sunlight possesses no special curative powers. We now know that it *cannot* cure or "dry up" colds. To the contrary, recent evidence demonstrates that it may worsen certain viral conditions. For example, ultraviolet light exposure can trigger outbreaks of certain viral skin infections, such as herpes and warts (see Chapter 5).

The sun also cannot cure acne. While many people do find that their acne blemishes "dry" up in the sun, unhappily, many of these same individuals observe the appearance of numerous small whiteheads about four to six weeks later. These whiteheads result from ultraviolet radiation-induced clogging of pores below the skin surface. Finally, the sun isn't even needed to supply our vitamin D needs. Actually, most people, except those in developing countries, get enough vitamin D through the foods they eat.

Unfortunately, despite all the recent publicity about the dangers of sunbathing, some people still remain unconvinced or refuse to be convinced. Others say, "I know it's bad for me, but I just can't give it up." Still others take an it's-not-going-to-happen-to-me attitude. Brochures about the sun, which can frequently be found in dermatologists' offices, are appropriately entitled: TAN NOW, PAY LATER, SUNTAN MINUS SUNBURN STILL EQUALS SUN DAMAGE, and TODAY'S HANDSOME TAN IS TOMORROW'S WRINKLE AND SKIN CANCER.

While a suntan eventually fades after the summer is over, the damage to skin from sunlight never does; sun damage is irreversible. In other words, every additional minute you spend suntanning results in one more minute of permanent skin damage. Remember, every time you see someone with a "healthy-looking" golden tan, you are looking at someone who has not only permanently damaged his or her skin but is at greater risk for the development of skin cancers.

Skin Types. You are probably already aware that some people seem to be more sensitive to the sun than others. Dermatologists group people into six skin types according to how sensitive they are to sun exposure (Table 1.1). Individuals with Types I and II skin tan poorly and are most prone to sunburn and other forms of sun damage. Most frequently, people with Types I or II skin are blondes or redheads having blue eyes who are of Irish or Northern European descent. Persons having Type V or VI skin are the least sensitive to the sun's effects. They usually tan deeply and seldom sunburn. Very dark-skinned Caucasians, Indians, and blacks usually fall into these two categories. Types III and IV are in between. Naturally, the lighter your skin color, the more cautious you must be about sun exposure.

Sensible Sun Exposure. Since it's clear that the sun is no good for you, what can you do to protect yourself? Of course, one possible answer is never to go out into the sun again. For most of us that would neither be practical nor desirable. Therefore, some general guidelines for sun sense and safety are in order:

1. Always use a strong sunscreen when outdoors between mid-April and mid-October, especially if you have Type I or Type II skin. Sunscreens are rated for efficiency by a number referred to as their *sun protection factor* (SPF). In general, for maximum safety, choose maximum protection sunscreens having an SPF of 15 or greater. An SPF of 15 means that if, for example, it would take you twenty minutes to become sunburned without using a sunscreen, it would take approximately fifteen times twenty minutes, or five hours, to become sunburned when using it. If you have especially oily skin or acne, you are

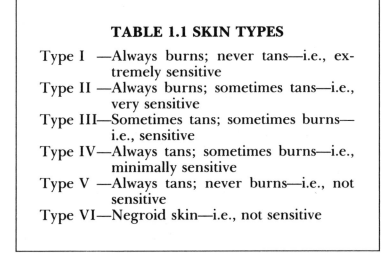

TABLE 1.1 SKIN TYPES

Type I —Always burns; never tans—i.e., extremely sensitive

Type II —Always burns; sometimes tans—i.e., very sensitive

Type III—Sometimes tans; sometimes burns—i.e., sensitive

Type IV—Always tans; sometimes burns—i.e., minimally sensitive

Type V —Always tans; never burns—i.e., not sensitive

Type VI—Negroid skin—i.e., not sensitive

better off choosing an alcohol-based sunscreen, such as **Presun, Tiscreen, Solbar PF, Solbar Plus,** or **Total Eclipse,** all with an SPF of 15. People with naturally darker complexions can use lower-numbered SPF sunscreens, if they wish.

2. Reapply the sunscreen every two to three hours if you tend to sweat heavily or are exercising vigorously.

3. Wear a sunscreen even when swimming. Water is capable of transmitting ultraviolet light, and you can get a sunburn even if you stay entirely submerged. You should also reapply the sunscreen *without delay* after swimming.

4. Limit your outdoor activities during the hours of 10:00 A.M. to 3:00 P.M., when the sun is directly overhead and strongest.

5. Wear protective clothing, such as broad-brimmed hats and large sunglasses.

6. Gradually build up your tolerance to the sun during the first week of the season. Increase your time in the sun each day by one-third of the previous day's exposure time. Don't use sun

reflectors; they concentrate the sun's damaging effects.

7. Don't be fooled into believing that sitting under a shade tree, beach umbrella, or boardwalk is adequate protection; 60 to 80 percent of the sun's rays can be reflected by sand and water.
8. Use sunscreens when skiing; snow also reflects the sun's rays.
9. Don't be fooled by a cloudy day; many of the sun's ultraviolet rays can pass through the clouds and give you a severe sunburn.
10. *Don't* use sunlamps or go to tanning salons. Ultraviolet light emitted from artificial sources may be more concentrated and thus potentially even more damaging than that from the sun.

Skin Cleansing

Proper skin cleansing is the second most important aspect of keeping your skin healthy. Two important rules apply: 1) Don't waste your money buying any soap that claims to do more for you than help you clean your skin. 2) To reduce the chance of overdryness and irritation, *don't* massage a soap into your skin. Lather up quickly and immediately and rinse off.

The main reasons for washing are to remove dirt, cosmetics, oils, bacteria, dead skin cells, and perspiration—and nothing more. Soaps and detergents merely help to dissolve grease and grime so that they may be easily washed away with water. Soaps cannot cure acne and they cannot give you perfect skin. But they can help you to feel fresher and cleaner.

Toilet Soaps. A toilet soap is merely a skin cleanser derived from animal or vegetable fats. Plain toilet soaps can work well for most people who have normal or oily skin. However, they tend to be a little more alkaline and drying than some of the milder soaps and cleansers discussed next. After more than a hundred years, **Ivory** soap still remains the industry standard. In general, toilet soaps are inexpensive and clean satisfactorily.

Soaps Containing Special Additives. As a rule, soaps containing special added ingredients cost more but do nothing more for you. These soaps may contain fruit, vegetable, and herbal extracts. None of these added ingredients is of any proven benefit to your skin. Abrasive soaps, which contain fine abrasive particles, also do not provide any significant benefits. In fact, they tend to be too irritating for many people. So-called medicated acne soaps do contain beneficial ingredients such as sulfur, salicylic acid, and benzoyl peroxide. However, when incorporated into a soap, these ingredients do little because they are rinsed off your skin before they have a chance to start working (see Chapter 4). In addition, acne soaps are often unnecessarily drying and irritating, especially for people with naturally sensitive skin.

Mild Skin Cleansers. If you have dry or chapped skin, or if you are being treated for acne with drying or peeling agents (see Chapter 4), you may find regular toilet soap too drying or irritating for regular use. A variety of milder soaps and cleansers are commercially available. These include superfatted soaps, transparent soaps, soapless soaps, and washable creams and lotions. As a rule, each of these types of soaps and cleansers seems to do a good job of gently cleansing naturally dry or chapped skin. Which particular brand of cleanser you choose becomes a matter of how much you are willing to pay, as well as your personal preferences for the look, feel, or smell of each of these products.

Superfatted soaps contain extra amounts of oils and fats, such as lanolin, olive oil, cocoa butter, or cold cream, hence the name superfatted. **Purpose, Dove, Basis,** and **Oilatum** are examples of this type of soap. Some people dislike superfatted soaps, complaining that they leave a greasy residue on the skin.

Transparent soaps, so-called because they are clear, likewise have a higher fat content than plain toilet soap. They also include ingredients such as glycerin, alcohol, and sugar, which are responsible for their transparency and softness. **Neutrogena** soap is a well-known example of a transparent soap. Many people dislike the fact that transparent soaps melt easily in soap dishes.

Soapless soaps, also called detergent soaps, are synthetic soaps made from petroleum derivatives. They generally lather well and have been specifically formulated to be less drying and less alkaline. **Lowila** cake is an example of a soapless soap. Some people prefer soapless soaps because they do not leave a filmy residue on the skin after using them. As an added advantage, these soaps are not affected by hard water. Magnesium and calcium salts in hard water are responsible for causing ordinary soaps to leave a residue of soap scum on your skin, as well as in the basin.

Finally, washable creams and lotions are particularly useful for people with naturally very dry, easily irritated skin. Washable creams and lotions are basically moisturizing lotions to which soaps or detergents have been added. These cleansers are also useful for people with certain skin conditions, such as eczema or psoriasis (see Chapter 5). **Cetaphil** lotion and **Phresh 3.5** lotion are excellent examples of washable lotions.

Deodorant Soaps. Deodorant soaps are toilet soaps to which antibacterial chemicals have been added for suppressing the growth of odor-producing bacteria on your skin. For this reason, they are also called *antibacterial* soaps. Deodorants frequently also contain fragrances for masking odor. Since facial skin contains no odor-producing sweat glands, and since deodorant soaps may be overly drying for the face, use them on the body only. **Safeguard** and **Dial** are examples of effective deodorant soaps.

Moisturizers

The function of moisturizers is not to add moisture to your skin but to smooth and soften it and lock in its natural moisture. Moisturizers are frequently also referred to as *lubricants* or *emollients*. Despite what some of you may have read or heard to the contrary, under ordinary circumstances, most young people do not need to use moisturizers at all. In fact, the routine use of thick, creamy moisturizers can make your skin unnecessarily oily, clog your pores, and aggravate acne.

Available as creams or lotions, moisturizers are helpful, however, for softening and soothing naturally dry or sensitive skin. Moisturizers can also be useful for offsetting the undesirable overdrying, irritating, or peeling effects of many topical acne remedies. Finally, they are particularly useful for skin protection during wet, cold, chapping weather.

If you need a moisturizer, choose an oil-free or water-based one. These are less likely to clog pores and aggravate acne. You should avoid oil-based moisturizers, as well as those that contain known acne-aggravating ingredients. Moreover, it is recommended that you use lotions rather than creams, particularly for use on the face. Lotions are simply creams to which more water has been added. Lotions are usually lighter, less thick, and go on more smoothly. Many people dislike the more greasy feel of thick creams.

Table 1.2 lists some of the most common ingredients contained in moisturizers according to their likelihood for aggravating acne. In general, if you are acne-prone, you should avoid products containing petrolatum (petroleum jelly), heavy mineral oil, and lanolin. These ingredients can be particular troublemakers. **Moisturel, Aquacare, U-Lactin, Lacticare,** and **Nutraderm** are effective moisturizers that have been found not to aggravate acne.

Finally, be sceptical of advertised claims for the supposed health benefits of certain added ingredients. The following ingredients when included in a moisturizer are of doubtful value: Vitamin E, collagen, proteins, elastin, amino acids, hormones, hyaluronic acid, RNA, aloe vera, algae, allantoin, placental extract, eggs, milk, and honey. Their inclusion in moisturizers, however, often adds considerably to the price of the products that contain them.

TABLE 1.2 MOISTURIZING
INGREDIENTS AND ACNE

Avoid	OK to Use
Isopropyl myristate	Octyl palmitate
Isopropyl esters	Isostearyl neopentate
Oleic acid	Cottonseed oil
Steric acid	Corn oil
Petrolatum	Safflower oil
Lanolin	Propylene glycol
Heavy mineral oil	Light mineral oil
Acetylated lanolin alcohols	Spermacetti
Lanolin fatty acid	Beeswax
Linseed oil	Sodium lauryl sulfate
Olive oil	
Cocoa butter	

Effects of Nutrition, Exercise,
and Stress on Your Skin

Your life-style—the way you live—can dramatically affect your apearance. What you eat, what you drink, and what you feel can make big differences in the way you look. After sun exposure, the three remaining cardinal sins against both your general health and the health of your skin are smoking, alcohol, and drugs.

Nutrition. Vitamins are organic substances, and minerals are inorganic substances. Both are essential for running and fueling the metabolic processes in your body. To date, thirteen vitamins and more than sixteen essential minerals have been identified. The vitamins A, C, and D, and the minerals iron, zinc, and calcium are well-known and much-written-about substances essential for many aspects of continued good health.

Unquestionably, deficiencies of certain vitamins and minerals can adversely affect your general health and appearance. As an example, severe vitamin C deficiency can result in easy bruisability and fragile, bleeding gums. Other examples include severe deficiencies of vitamin B_6, or niacin, which can lead to various types of skin rashes. However, despite what health food stores and vitamin and mineral manufacturers would like you to believe, most people consuming ordinary Western diets, even those who live on fast food or junk food diets, do not usually become vitamin or mineral deficient. Under ordinary circumstances, most Americans do not need vitamin or mineral supplements.

Finally, vitamins and minerals have not been proven, as some people mistakenly believe, to possess any magical or curative powers. Taking daily vitamin and mineral supplements cannot stop you from feeling nervous, help you feel less run-down, make up for a lack of sleep, or cure the common cold. They also cannot make you more beautiful or a better athlete. In general, it is not harmful to take multivitamin and mineral supplements on a daily basis, so long as you do not exceed the Food and Drug Administration's (FDA) recommended daily allowances (RDA) for them. However, since the mineral iodine can aggravate acne, acne sufferers should avoid mineral supplements containing iodine. Naturally, if you have any specific questions about proper nutrition, ask your doctor.

Exercise. Regular exercise is good, both for your general health and for your skin. Working out can improve your skin's color and texture by increasing blood flow. Increased blood flow means the delivery of more oxygen and nutrients to your skin, and this accounts, in large measure, for that healthy "glow" seen after a good workout. In addition, the increased muscle tone and weight control, which frequently accompany a regular exercise program, further contribute to improving overall appearance and well-being.

Exercising is not without its problems, however. On the down side, regular, vigorous exercise can subject your skin directly and indirectly to quite a beating.

Regardless of what types of exercises or vigorous activities you pursue, your skin acts as a barrier between you and the outside world. As a result, it can be subjected to a variety of abuses, including sun, wind, water, heat, cold, scrapes, bruises, blisters, and the effects of excessive sweating.

By taking a few simple precautions, you can prevent problems and enjoy yourself more. The importance of sun protection, skin cleansing, and moisturizing has already been discussed. These three areas become even more important when you exercise regularly. In addition, you should remove any makeup before exercising, to permit better sweat evaporation from your skin. Remove your jewelry, as well. Jewelry may not only get in the way of your workout but can be responsible for causing allergies and irritation. Costume jewelry, and even gold jewelry, contains some nickel. In nickel-sensitive persons, problems result when small amounts of nickel are leached out of their jewelry by heavy perspiration. If your jewelry absolutely must be worn during exercise, dust it lightly with some talcum powder to keep the skin areas under it dry.

No matter which sports or exercises you enjoy, you should always try to wear the proper clothing and protective gear for your activity. In general, in warm weather, wear loose, light clothing. Loose weaves, such as cotton, rather than synthetics, permit better sweat evaporation. In cold weather, dress in layers. Wearing layers of clothing not only provides you with better insulation but permits you to remove individual layers as you warm up.

Finally, exercise wear should be changed and laundered *after each use*. You should wash your clothes in a gentle detergent, such as **Ivory Snow**, to reduce the buildup of odor and potentially skin-irritating bacteria. Harsh detergents and fabric softeners should generally be avoided since they can irritate your skin if leached out of your exercise clothing by sweat.

Stress. Many skin conditions can be aggravated or triggered by increased nervous tension. These include such common conditions as acne, profuse sweating, facial flushing, itching, certain allergies, eczema, and psoriasis (see Chapter 5). Interestingly, as an illustration of the power of mind over matter, warts have been known to suddenly disappear when children have been convinced by their doctors that a placebo (fake) wart remedy was really a powerful medication.

The effects of our emotions and stress on our skin is only now beginning to be really appreciated. In certain circumstances, doctors are even starting to recommend the use of relaxation and meditation, in addition to the use of conventional medical therapies, for some of their patients with certain skin conditions. However, before any concrete recommendations can be made, much remains to be learned about our "emotional skin" and how we can best deal with the effects of our emotions on our skin.

Effects of Smoking, Alcohol, and Drugs

Smoking, heavy drinking, or drugs can wreck your skin and your health in general. The life-threatening consequences of smoking, namely emphysema, lung cancer, and heart disease, have been well publicized and are probably well known to you. However, cigarette smoking can have serious effects on your skin as well (Fig. 1.2). Age for age, studies indicate that heavy smokers have sallower, more wrinkled skin than nonsmokers. Cigarette-related facial skin changes have been referred to as the "smoker's face." These changes may be due, at least in part, to the constricting effects of nicotine or other cigarette smoke byproducts on the small blood vessels in the skin. Although publicity about the heart and lung hazards of cigarette smoking has not as yet stemmed the tide of cigarette smoking, perhaps greater awareness that it can cause severe wrinkling, sagging, and aging of the skin will.

Light drinking has not been shown to be necessarily unhealthy for the skin. This, of course, does not mean that it is healthy for you, either. On the other hand, heavy drinking, among its other physically and psychologically damaging effects, can lead to excessive facial

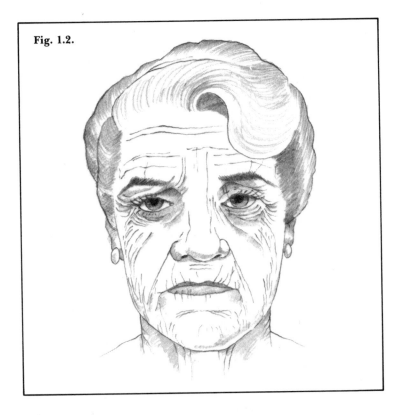

"Smoker's Face"
Wrinkles radiate from the upper and lower lips
and from the corners of the eyes. The cheeks
are deeply lined and there are numerous
shallow lines on the cheeks and lower jaw.

flushing, owing to dilation of the small blood vessels in the skin. After many years of repeated flushing episodes in certain predisposed individuals, the tiny blood vessels can lose their ability to constrict, resulting in the formation of a dense network of disfiguring reddish-purplish marks over the cheeks and nose. Furthermore, alcohol damage to the liver can lead to the formation of other kinds of blood vessel abnormalities on other parts of the body, as well. In short, excessive alcohol can ruin not only your life but your looks.

All drugs with abuse potential, including the so-called recreational drugs, have been associated with ill effects on the skin. Tranquilizers and "downers" can cause allergic reactions resulting in skin-shedding. Barbiturates can cause blisters around the mouth and on the hips and ankles. "Uppers" ("speed," amphetamines, cocaine) can cause severely dry, chapped lips and allergic rashes. Marijuana ("pot," "joints") can cause hives and "pinkeye" and may aggravate acne. It has even been associated with instances of hair loss. Amyl nitrites, ("rush," "poppers," "sniffers"), by interfering with the proper oxygenation of the skin, can temporarily give it a bluish coloration. Glue sniffing can irritate and peel the skin around the nose and cause oozing. Cocaine sniffing can lead to perforation of the cartilage in the nose, leaving a hole between the nostrils. Heroin abuse can result in ulcers, clots, infections, and scars at injection sites; in addition, heroin addicts typically appear older and more wrinkled. Chronic heroin abuse has been linked with loss of skin elasticity and the formation of dark circles and rings around the eyes. In short, drugs and alcohol can wreck your appearance and your life. If you have an alcohol or drug problem, seek help before it's too late. If you don't drink, or haven't done drugs, don't start.

2

The Makeup of Cosmetics

Without a doubt, the manufacture and sale of cosmetics are big business. More than $1.5 billion is spent annually on cosmetics, largely by women, and this figure is expected to continue to grow at a rapid rate. Cosmetics are technically defined as products that are intended to make you look better. By contrast, medications applied to the skin (doctors call them *topical medications*) are defined as products that affect the structure or function of your skin. Although topical medications are subject to strict FDA regulation, cosmetics are not. Thus, the burden of wisely choosing cosmetics falls largely on you, the consumer.

Both the enormous variety of cosmetics available and their variations in price can make choosing the right cosmetics difficult. Literally scores of different types of cosmetics are available for use on every area of your skin, hair, and nails. Moreover, different brands of cosmetics intended for the same purposes, often containing the same or very similar active ingredients, may vary in cost from pennies to tens of dollars for equal amounts. To make matters worse, advertisers actively compete to make their products sound like the answer to your prayers, often making wild, too-good-to-be-true claims for their products' benefits.

Happily, the FDA requires that all American cosmetic manufacturers list their products' ingredients on the label. They are also required to list those ingredients in the order of their relative amounts in the product. In other words, a particular cosmetic will contain more of those ingredients listed first on the label and less of those listed last. It almost goes without saying that by knowing something about what and how much of an ingredient goes into a particular cosmetic, you will be better equipped to make the right purchases.

Unfortunately, cosmetic ingredient labels can themselves often be confusing and occasionally misleading. For example, to protect product manufacturers from having to divulge certain trade secrets or secret formulas, cosmetic manufacturers are not required to list the names of such items as the specific fragrances or flavorings in their products. They also need not list the precise amounts of any of the ingredients in them. Moreover, the current law permits ingredients to be listed according to either their common, chemical, or trade names. Thus, one company may list an ingredient by its chemical name and another company will list that same ingredient by its common name. This creates unnecessary confusion. Because of this confusion with ingredient names, comparing products to see if they contain the same ingredients can sometimes be very difficult.

It would seem that being a smart consumer is an almost impossible job, requiring knowledge of advanced cosmetic chemistry. This is not the case. With a little background information, you can purchase cosmetics more knowledgeably and even save money. In this chapter, you will learn a new approach to reading a cosmetic label. You will also learn what goes into your favorite makeups, which product ingredient claims not to be fooled by, and what to watch out for. A table of common cosmetic ingredients and their functions is also included, to make it easier for you to examine product labels.

ADVERTISING BUZZ WORDS
TO WATCH OUT FOR

Although federal agencies exist to police advertisers and prevent them from making distorted or downright phony claims, these agencies simply do not have enough staff to do an adequate job. As a result, you have to watch out for yourself. Whenever you read an advertisement or see or hear a commercial, you should be on your guard for certain words or phrases that advertisers love to use to hook you into buying their products. These words or phrases should make you immediately sceptical: *amazing, fantastic, miraculous, remarkable, exciting, instant-acting, fast-acting, revolutionary, works wonders, vanishing,* and *guaranteed.* Medical-sounding advertising phrases include: *breakthrough, medically approved, doctor-tested, independent laboratory-tested, secret formula, European or Oriental formula, amazing discovery, clinical, natural, herbal, organic, special technology,* and *secret know-how.*

To repeat, any product that sounds too good to be true most likely is.

THE INGREDIENTS
IN COSMETICS

The major trick to being a better consumer is knowing which ingredients in a product do something to benefit you and which are there to either preserve the product or benefit the product manufacturer. Those ingredients in a cosmetic put there to help you can be called the *active ingredients.* Those ingredients needed to manufacture a product, or preserve it from spoiling, can be referred to as the *inactive ingredients.* Those ingredients that have no proven value but have been included to increase sales appeal or advertising hype can be labeled *exotic additives.*

Being able to separate the active from the inactive and exotic ingredients in any cosmetic has tremendous practical value. For example, when looking to buy a moisturizer, clearly, the active ingredients are the moisturizing ingredients that serve to soften and smooth your skin. In the case of foundation makeups, for example, both the pigments (colors) and the moisturizing base constitute the active ingredients. The pigment gives you the color and shade that you want and the moisturizing base allows the colors to be applied smoothly and evenly.

Solvents, emulsifying agents, emulsion stabilizers, viscosity builders, preservatives, antioxidants, and thickening, stiffening, and suspending agents are all forms of inactive ingredients. These tongue-twisting groups of ingredients basically keep a product stable, blend its individual ingredients, and retard spoilage, but they don't directly do anything for your appearance. Exotic ingredients—frequently of unproven value or downright useless—may be added to a cosmetic to generate greater appeal and higher prices. You can see, then, that to make life simpler for yourself when deciding between several products used for the same purpose, you need only to compare their active ingredients. You can basically ignore the inactive and exotic ingredients.

Table 2.1 can be used to help you separate active from inactive and exotic ingredients when purchasing an item. To make the table more comprehensible, a few simple definitions are in order. Emollients, as you may recall from Chapter 1, are chemicals used to soften and smooth your skin. Humectants are substances that absorb moisture from the air and also lock in moisture in the skin. Solvents, the best example of which is plain water, are carrier liquids into which other ingredients are dissolved. Emulsifying agents help oil and water stay mixed in lotions and creams. Emulsion stabilizers keep oil and water from separating. Preservatives, antioxidants, and chemical stabilizers prolong shelf life by suppressing germs and preventing unwanted chemical reactions. Viscosity builders and thickening, stiffening,

TABLE 2.1 COMMON COSMETIC INGREDIENTS BY FUNCTION

Emollients
Butyl stearate
Caprylic/capric triglyceride
Castor oil
Cetearyl alcohol
Cetyl alcohol
Diisopropyl adipate
Glycerin
Glyceryl monostearate
Isopropyl myristate
Isopropyl palmitate
Lanolin
Lanolin alcohol
Lanolin, hydrogenated
Mineral oil
Petrolatum
Polyethylene glycols
Polyoxethylene lauryl ether
Polyoxypropylene 15 stearyl ether
Propylene glycol stearate
Silicone
Squalane
Stearic acid
Stearyl alcohol
Vegetable oils

Humectants
Glycerin
Lactic acid

Humectants
(cont.)
Lecithin
Propylene glycol
Sorbitol solution
Urea

Solvents
Alcohol
Diisopropyl adipate
Glycerin
1,2,6-hexanetriol
Isopropyl myristate
Polyoxypropylene 15 stearyl ether
Propylene carbonate
Propylene glycol

Emulsifying agents
(Surfactants)
Amphoteric-9
Carbomer
Cetearyl alcohol (and) ceteareth-20
Cholesterol
Disodium monooleamidosulfosuccinate
Emulsifying wax, NF
Lanolin
Lanolin alcohol (Laureths)
Lanolin, hydrogenated
Lecithin

TABLE 2.1 (cont.)

Emulsifying agents (cont.)
Polyethylene (*Surfactants*) 1000 monocetyl ether
Polyoxyl 40 stearate
Polysorbates
Sodium laureth sulfate
Sodium lauryl sulfate
Sorbitan esters
Stearic acid
TEA stearate
Trolamine

Emulsion stabilizers and viscosity builders
Carbomer
Cetearyl alcohol
Cetyl alcohol
Glyceryl monostearate
Paraffin
Polyethylene glycols
Propylene glycol stearate
Stearyl alcohol

Preservatives, antioxidants, and chemical stabilizers
Alcohol
Benzyl alcohol
Butylated hydroxyanisole (BHA)
Butylated hydroxytoluene (BHT)

Preservatives, antioxidants and chemical stabilizers (cont.)
Chlorocresol
Citric acid
Edetate disodium
EDTA
Imidazolidinyl urea
Parabens
Phenyl mercuric acetate
Potassium sorbate
Propyl gallate
Propylene glycol
Quarternium-15
Sodium bisulfite
Sorbic acid
Tocopherol (vitamin E)

Thickening, stiffening, and suspending agents
Beeswax
Candelill wax
Carbomer
Carnauba wax
Cellulose gums
Cetyl esters wax
Dextrin
Mannitol
Ozokerite (Ceresin)
Polyethylene
Xanthan gum

Gellants
Carbomer

TABLE 2.1 (cont.)

Gellants (cont.)
Carboxymethyl cellulose
Hydroxymethyl cellulose
Methyl cellulose

Powder formers
Magnesium aluminum
  silicate
Magnesium silicate
Talc

Common pigments
(colors)
Bismuth oxychloride
  (pearlizers)
Carmine
Chromium oxide
Ferric ammonium ferrocyanide
Ferric ferrocyanide
Iron oxide

Common pigments
(colors) (cont.)
Manganese violet
Mica (pearlizers)
Ultramarine blue

Exotic ingredients
(additives of unproven
value)
Algae
Allantoin
Aloe vera
Collagen
Eggs
Elastin
Honey
Hyaluronic acid
Milk
Placental extract
RNA
Vitamin A
Vitamin E
  (tocopherol)

and suspending agents are used to give a "cushiony" feel to products and to thicken their consistency. Gellants are special kinds of thickeners that, when combined with alcohol, acetone, or water, make transparent gels. Powder formers, as their name implies, are used to formulate powdery products. Finally, in the complex world of cosmetic chemistry, many ingredients serve more than one purpose.

By now, it should be obvious that a cosmetic displaying a label bearing a long list of ingredients with impressive chemical names is not necessarily better than its competitors. Except for astringents and perfumes, you will find that the basic formulas for the overwhelming majority of most commonly used facial cosmetics are merely variations upon the old cold cream (moisturizer) formula, to which pigments or other special active ingredients have been added for particular purposes.

MOISTURIZERS

Moisturizers, as you already learned in Chapter 1, are cosmetics intended to smooth and soften skin and lock in its natural water content. Modified in one way or another to meet a particular need—sometimes just a little, sometimes dramatically—moisturizers are the bases for most of the other types of cosmetics discussed.

As said above, all moisturizer formulas are basically variations of the formula for cold cream: water, waxes, oils, or fats. They are available as lotions or creams. As a rule, oil-free or water-based moisturizers contain more water and less oil. As a consequence, oil-free moisturizers are better for oily or acne-prone skin. Oil-based moisturizers, by contrast, contain less water and more oil. These moisturizers are better for dry or sensitive skin but tend to be acne-provoking. Nowadays, humectants such as lactic acid are frequently added to the basic moisturizer formula to increase its effectiveness.

MASKS AND PACKS

There are basically two types of masks: cream masks and paste masks. (You may find the word *mask* occasionally spelled *masque*.) Although of doubtful value, both cream and paste masks are supposed to absorb oil and promote mild peeling, while they cleanse and refresh your skin.

Cream masks have the basic oil, wax, and water formula of moisturizers. As such, they may aggravate oily or acne-prone skin. Paste masks, on the other hand, are composed of a powdery base to which abrasives such as almond meal, bran, oats, or ground apricot pits have been added. Bentonite, kaolin (Fuller's Earth), or magnesium aluminum silicate are used to thicken these products and enhance their ability to absorb oils. For some people with naturally sensitive skin or those being treated with drying acne medications, abrasive paste masks may be overly irritating.

In general, neither of these masks is recommended by dermatologists. Regular gentle soap and water cleansing is sufficient for removing oils, dirt, and cosmetics.

FOUNDATION MAKEUPS

Foundations are used to add evenness to skin tone and, if desired, to act as a base for blushes and eye makeups. In their simplest form, foundations are moisturizers to which pigments have been added to give them color; here both the pigments and the moisturizer can be considered the active ingredients. Oil-free foundations should be used by acne-prone individuals. Iron oxides and ultramarine blue are examples of common foundation pigments. Bismuth oxychloride and mica, called *pearlizers,* may also be added to impart a shimmering, glittering look. Finally, magnesium aluminum silicate or talc may be added to give a matte finish.

Masking cosmetics for covering up scars, skin discolorations, or other irregularities, very much like thick theater makeup, are simply heavy, water-resistant, oil-based foundations containing greater amounts of pigment for better coverage. Coversticks are thick, water-resistant foundations in stick form. They are primarily used to cover spot discolorations or irregularities. Coversticks generally contain a higher proportion of waxes for thickness and body.

BLUSHES

Blushes are cosmetics that are used to add color to the face and to provide shading and contour. Blushes are available in cream or powder forms. Cream blushes, like foundations, are composed simply of pigments supended in a thick, creamy, moisturizing base. For that reason, cream blushes tend to clog pores. You should avoid them if you are acne-prone. On the other hand, powder blushes are powder-based cosmetics to which pigments have been added. Powder blushes, because they are oil absorbent, are less likely to aggravate acne.

EYE SHADOWS

Eye shadows are used to provide color, highlights, and shading to the upper eyelids. Eye shadows, like blushes, come in liquid and powder forms. Liquid eye shadows are simply pigments in an oil/wax moisturizing base; powder shadows contain pigments suspended in a talc-rich, oil/wax-based moisturizer. The absence of water makes these products less likely to run. Pearlizers may be added to create a glittery, shimmery look.

EYELINERS

Eyeliners serve to emphasize and define the eyelids. They are sold in liquid and pencil form. Liquid eyeliners are made of wax/oil bases to which pigments and plasticizing chemicals, frequently acrylics or acrylates, have been added to impart luster and give body. Pencil eyeliners generally contain more wax for stiffening the eyeliner into pencil form.

Special care must be taken in applying and handling eyeliners. If applied improperly, too close to the lid margins or too close to the inner eyelids, eyeliner pigments may cause a chemical inflammation of the delicate mucous membranes on the inside of the eyelid. If granules of pigment embed themselves into the delicate eyelid membranes, they may permanently tattoo them. In addition, in order to prevent possible eye irritations, the concentrations of preservatives in eyeliners are purposely kept low. For this reason, special care should also be taken not to contaminate these products. To be safe, you should never share eye cosmetics with anyone else.

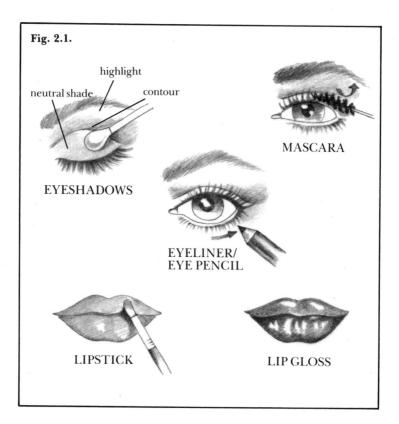

Fig. 2.1.

highlight

neutral shade   contour

EYESHADOWS

MASCARA

EYELINER/
EYE PENCIL

LIPSTICK

LIP GLOSS

Eye and Lip Cosmetics

MASCARAS

Mascaras are used to add color, definition, and intensity to eyelashes. They are sold in cake and liquid forms. Cake mascara is largely composed of a thick, water-free, oil/wax base to which the desired pigments are added. Cake mascaras are applied with a brush. Liquid mascaras contain heavy, oil-based moisturizing bases. Acrylates and shellacs are usually added to thicken mascaras and prevent running. Both types of mascaras need to be removed with soap and water or oil-based mineral cleansing lotions. Mascaras will not cause eyelashes to fall out, as some people needlessly fear, although loose hairs do come out when mascara is applied or removed. These hairs grow back.

Lash extender mascaras are simply liquid mascaras to which synthetic fibers, usually rayon, are added. These fibers coat your natural lashes and "extend" them. People with contact lenses should avoid lash extender mascaras. If these synthetic fibers get under contact lenses, corneal scratching or more severe corneal damage can result.

LIPSTICKS AND LIP GLOSSES

Lipsticks add color to your lips, and lip glosses add shine. These cosmetics share a basic oil/wax base. In the case of lipsticks, pigments are added to impart color; in the case of glosses, sheen-producing ingredients, such as lanolin, are added. Sunscreens, such as PABA or its derivatives, are frequently added to lipsticks to protect lips from excessive sun damage. The addition of fragrances and flavorings to lip glosses provides no additional benefits. They constitute useless and exotic additives.

ASTRINGENTS, FRESHENERS, AND TONERS

Intended to "freshen and cleanse" skin and "shrink" pores, these types of cosmetics do little more than make your face feel cool, tight, and tingly. All three types are basically composed of water, alcohol, and fragrances. Interestingly, colognes and perfumes share the same basic water, alcohol, and fragrance formula. However, colognes and perfumes contain less alcohol and more fragrance.

For naturally dry, sensitive skin, or for people being treated with drying, antiacne medications, astringents can be irritating, particularly if used during the winter months. Even for people with oily skin, a soap and water cleansing is all that is usually necessary. The addition of witch hazel, menthol, or camphor to these products may add a tingly sensation but little else. For fragrance, mint, eucalyptus, and lemon may be added, but these confer no special properties. Some people with excessively oily skin, especially during hot, humid weather, may find astringents helpful for blotting up oiliness. But even under those circumstances, astringents should be used infrequently because they tend to overdry and irritate.

HYPOALLERGENIC COSMETICS

Allergies to cosmetics may show up as redness, itching, swelling, and blistering. Fortunately, true allergic reactions to cosmetics are rare. Allergic individuals and people with very sensitive skin often look for products labeled *hypoallergenic*. Contrary to what you may think, the term hypoallergenic does not mean that a particular product cannot cause an allergic reaction. It only means that a cosmetic manufacturer has taken measures to exclude certain types of ingredients, such as perfumes and fragrances, which are known to have a greater likelihood of causing allergies. And should you have an allergic reaction, those companies producing hypoallergenic products are more likely to help your dermatologist in any way possible to find the ingredient(s) in their product that may be causing the problem. They will often provide your doctor with a complete list of ingredients and may also supply sample amounts of these ingredients in a form for allergy testing.

Whether a product is labeled hypoallergenic or not, most major cosmetic manufacturers produce basically hypoallergenic products. If for no other reason, it makes good business sense. Think about it. Companies are in business to sell products and make money. No company is going to be so unmindful as to deliberately manufacture a product that has such a strong likelihood of causing allergic reactions that many people would be forced to stop using it.

If you suspect that you have an allergy to any cosmetic, immediately discontinue using it. Once the allergic reaction subsides, you should choose another brand of cosmetic. If no problem develops with the new brand, you may continue to use it. On the other hand, if you continue to have allergic problems, see your dermatologist. He or she has a variety of means, including the use of painless allergy tests, called *patch tests*, for finding out which ingredients may be causing your problem.

3

The Acne Problem

Few skin problems can be more disturbing than having pimples, or "zits." Dermatologists call this *acne vulgaris.* That's because pimples usually strike where they can be most plainly seen—the face, neck, chest, and back.

Most people suffer with acne at some time in their lives, even if it's no more than the occasional appearance of an isolated blemish. However, teenagers are more prone to acne than other age groups, which is the reason that ordinary acne is commonly referred to as "teenage acne." More than 80 percent of adolescents will develop acne to some extent, and nearly 95 percent of the population will suffer from acne to some degree at some time in their lives. Acne is an old problem that, as far as we know, has been plaguing people since the dawn of time.

Because acne is such a highly visible problem, it frequently causes much needless psychological suffering, embarrassment, and loss of self-esteem. Even worse, severe acne, if untreated or treated improperly, can result in permanent, disfiguring scars, and these may remain a lifelong source of embarrassment. Occasionally, thoughtless comments by friends or relatives can make matters worse. Some adults consider teenage acne to be a kind of semihumorous skin problem, an awkward phase that every young person has to go through as part of growing up. Teasing and taunting names such as "pizza face," even made in jest by peers or siblings, can be further sources of humiliation, loss of self-confidence, and social withdrawal. As any sufferer can tell you, pimples are no laughing matter.

Even though pimples have been around for thousands of years and are such a common problem, doctors still lack many answers about what causes them. They also do not know all the steps in their formation. Fortunately, however, much is already known about acne, and many successful treatments are available (see Chapter 4). Not surprisingly, therefore, acne sufferers make up a large percentage of the patients seen by most dermatologists in their private practices.

Many myths and misconceptions surround acne and its causes. The remainder of this chapter is devoted to exploring the causes of acne and exploding some of the more common myths surrounding it.

OILY SKIN

Even when acne itself is not much of a problem, many people complain of having excessively shiny and oily skin. Male hormones, called *androgens*—produced following puberty *both* in boys and, to a lesser extent, in girls—are responsible for stimulating your oil glands to secrete. This is why oily skin and acne are seldom a problem before the onset of adolescence. Precisely because their glands secrete more male hormones, boys usually have more severe cases of acne than girls. Besides glandular secretion, other factors affect the oiliness of your skin. These include changes in your emotions, in outside temperature, and in the amount of sun exposure you receive. Interestingly, although the majority of acne sufferers have oily skin, you don't *have* to have oily skin to have acne. In fact, you can have very dry skin and have severe acne nonetheless.

HOW ACNE
BLEMISHES FORM

Nobody knows the exact cause(s) of acne. However, inheritance factors (genes) appear to play an important role. In other words, acne appears to run in certain families. If your parents have had acne, you are more likely to also. Racial factors also play a role; in general, white people tend to have more severe forms of acne than black people.

Most people mistakenly believe that acne is an infection of the skin. It isn't. Instead, it is what doctors refer to as an *inflammation* of the skin. An inflammation is any irritating condition that is accompanied by redness, tenderness, swelling, heat, and pain. An *infection,* on the other hand, is a form of inflammation caused by bacterial, fungal, or viral germs (see Chapter 5).

Figure 3.1 illustrates the structures composing a normal hair follicle and our current understanding of the basic steps in the development of pimples. As you can see, the acne-forming process begins within the hair follicles, or pores. Hair follicles are present on everyone's skin, although in most women, facial hairs can be so extremely fine as to be almost invisible to the naked eye. (You may be able to see these fine hairs if you look carefully at your face with a magnifying glass.) Acne primarily develops in those areas where your pores contain larger, more actively secreting oil glands. These areas include your face (particularly your chin, forehead, and cheeks), neck, back, chest, and shoulders.

Under normal circumstances, the outermost layer of dead cells lining your hair follicles is shed each day. These cells are "washed" to the surface of your skin by your oil-gland secretions. In those people having the inherited tendency to develop acne, the lining cells of the follicles not only seem to stick to each other more but appear to be shed in greater numbers. As a result, shed cells tend to clump together and, instead of being easily "washed" to the surface of your skin, begin to form plugs at or near the openings of your pores. *Open comedos,* or blackheads, are plugged follicles where

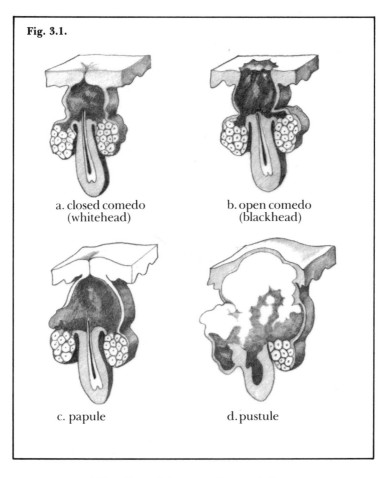

Fig. 3.1.

a. closed comedo
(whitehead)

b. open comedo
(blackhead)

c. papule

d. pustule

The Four Types of Blemishes

the plug rests within the opening of the pore and remains exposed to the skin surface. By contrast, *closed comedos,* or whiteheads, are plugged pores where the plug lies just beneath the skin surface. Although blackheads may be more unsightly, whiteheads, as you will soon see, are the true troublemakers. Whiteheads may best be thought of as small, potentially explosive packets of TNT resting under the skin. Whiteheads remain ready and waiting for the right stimuli to detonate them into potentially scarring pimples and cysts.

Since whiteheads are clogged pores with no openings to the skin surface, shed skin cells and oil-gland secretions within the follicles continue to accumulate. Bacteria called *Propionobacterium acnes,* which normally inhabit your pores, begin to break down the accumulating debris within the follicles into irritating substances called *fatty acids.* As the fatty acids and other debris continue to accumulate, the follicle walls continue to expand like balloons under the skin until they finally rupture and spill out their irritating contents into the surrounding skin. Acne pimples, pustules, and cysts are the result.

ACNE CAN BE SERIOUS

Acne blemishes can range from mild to severe. In order to help dermatologists select the appropriate treatment for each patient, they have developed a way of grading the severity of a person's acne condition:

Grade I (mild acne): People with grade I acne generally have blackheads and/or whiteheads; pimples are *not* present.

Grade II (moderate acne): Blackheads, whiteheads, and small pimples are present, but they are usually confined to the face; inflammation is minimal.

Grade III (severe acne): Blackheads, whiteheads, and deeper pimples are present; inflammation is more pronounced.

Grade IV (very severe): The outbreak is widespread and frequently involves the neck, shoulders, chest, and back. Many pustules and deeper cysts are found. Scarring is also frequently present.

FACTORS THAT
AGGRAVATE ACNE

You have just learned that acne begins as a tendency to form plugs at or near the openings of your pores, setting off a chain of events below the skin surface that leads to the formation of pimples, pustules, and cysts. If you have ever suffered with acne, you have probably already observed that there are times when your skin seems to improve by itself and other times when it flares up. Unfortunately, not all the factors triggering acne flare-ups are known. However, it is well established that various kinds of physical and emotional stresses can cause acne to worsen.

Although nervous tension is not a cause of acne, it appears in many people to play a very important role in aggravating it. The pressure of midterm or final exams, a blind date, prom night, a fight with your boyfriend or girlfriend, an argument with your parents, or a death in the family are all examples of stressful situations that have been known to result in acne flare-ups. The acne will frequently improve once the emotionally stressful period has passed.

Physical stresses on your body can also aggravate the acne condition. Having a cold, fever, sore throat, or allergy attack, for example, have all been associated with acne flare-ups. Premenstrual flare-ups are common, although some women experience acne breakouts during ovulation instead. In addition, certain medications used to treat epilepsy, tuberculosis, and emotional disorders may worsen a preexisting acne problem. So may the use of topical steroid creams. Interestingly, the birth control pill can worsen acne in some people but improve it in others.

Finally, oily liquids or thick creamy cosmetics are frequently acne-producing. The heavier the preparation, the more likely it is to contain acne-producing substances such as petroleum jelly, mineral oil, or lanolin derivatives. Greases of any kind, which may contaminate your skin, generally aggravate acne.

COMMON MYTHS AND MISCONCEPTIONS ABOUT ACNE

1. Acne is caused by dirt. This is one of the most common misconceptions. Acne is *not* caused by dirt.

Very likely, the dirtlike appearance of blackheads may have given rise to this misconception. Unfortunately, because acne is so often mistakenly associated with dirt, many acne sufferers are made to feel as though they are "dirty" people who don't wash enough. In actuality, the black substance in blackheads is *not* dirt. Rather, it is believed to be an oxidized skin pigment. More simply, it's a kind of skin "rust."

2. Superscrubbing and drying your skin will clear up acne. The myth linking acne and dirt, as well as the generally unwashed look of very oily skin, are most probably responsible for this belief, too. As you learned earlier, acne starts *below* the skin surface. Therefore, overscrubbing and overdrying the surface of your skin will do nothing useful for you. In fact, superscrubbing often may precipitate an acne breakout by rupturing whiteheads below the skin surface, releasing the irritating fatty acids and starting the whole process rolling. Furthermore, too frequent or too vigorous washing can so overdry and irritate the surface of your skin that it becomes too uncomfortable to apply any real acne medications. Unfortunately, most acne medications tend to leave your skin a shade on the dry side after use. If you combine their use with a misguided attempt to superscrub away your acne problem, you risk developing extreme skin chapping, cracking, and flaking.

3. Acne is caused by letting your hair rest on your forehead. "Get your hair off your forehead or you'll give yourself pimples" is a favorite gripe of many parents. In reality, the surface oils coating your hairs are of little significance in the development of pimples. The oils that do play a role are those trapped within the clogged pores beneath your skin. Of course, oily hair itself can be unattractive and harder to manage, but that is a separate issue.

4. Acne is caused by certain foods, such as chocolates, fried foods, and nuts. This is another myth that has become so ingrained in our culture that it is often hard to make people give it up. Acne is *not* caused nor aggravated by eating chocolates, fried food, colas, nuts, potato chips, candy, ice cream, or pizza. These foods are not particularly healthful for your heart and blood vessels, however, so it is advisable to avoid them for that reason.

For those who have grown up believing that food triggers acne, the emotional stress and guilt caused by eating these "forbidden fruits" can be so great that acne may worsen. Naturally, such individuals should refrain from eating those foods that they believe cause them a problem.

Foods containing high concentrations of iodine, such as shellfish, kelp, iodized table salts, and certain mineral supplements, may aggravate acne in some people. Try to reduce your intake of these foods and supplements, especially if they make up a large part of your diet.

5. Acne is improved by sun exposure. Many of you may have observed that a moderate amount of sun exposure temporarily helps to dry up some surface blemishes and that a deep tan can further mask persistent blemishes and discolorations. However, most people are unaware that overexposure to the sun may actually cause acne to worsen. The sun's ultraviolet rays are capable of damaging the openings to your pores, resulting in the formation of whiteheads and the beginning of the acne chain of events discussed earlier. The subsequent development of whiteheads and acne breakouts generally occurs about four to six weeks after sun exposure.

Finally, as you learned in Chapter 1, strong evidence exists linking chronic sun exposure to the development of premature skin aging and skin cancers. Any short-term benefits of sun exposure for acne must be balanced against the risk of developing these possible long-term consequences.

6. Acne is incurable. Although it is true that doctors still cannot cure the basic, underlying familial (hereditary) basis for acne, many advances for controlling and treating acne have been developed, particularly during the past decade. A wide variety of very effective topical medications (lotions, creams, and ointments) and oral medications (drugs and pills) are now available. What you can do to help yourself and what your dermatologist can do for you are the subjects of the next chapter.

4

Acne Treatments

In the last chapter, we looked at the causes of acne and various misconceptions surrounding it. In this chapter, we will look at what you can do for yourself to prevent and control acne and what your doctor can do for you.

ACNE SELF-TREATMENT:
FOLLOW THE RULES

Rule #1: When in doubt, don't take chances with your skin. Seek a dermatologist's help. If your problem is more than just oily skin or a few blackheads, whiteheads, or pimples, this is the first and most important rule. Permanent scarring can result from neglected or improperly treated acne, particularly if you have a moderately severe or very severe acne problem.

Rule #2: Don't overscrub your skin. A gentle soap-and-water cleansing once or twice daily, even if you have very oily skin, is all you generally need to keep your skin feeling and looking clean. Mild soaps, such as **Lowila, Purpose, Dove,** and **Neutrogena** are good

TABLE 4.1
GENERAL TIPS FOR SELF-HELP

1) When in doubt, or if your problem is severe, seek professional help.
2) Use mild soaps and don't overwash or overscrub your skin.
3) Use only oil-free moisturizers, oil-free or gel foundations, and powder or gel blushes.
4) Avoid astringents.
5) Avoid abrasive sponges or washcloths.
6) Don't pick, squeeze, or pop your pimples.

for this purpose. So-called acne soaps, abrasive soaps (those containing abrasive particles), alkaline soaps, and deodorants soaps should be avoided. They don't clean your skin any better, and they may make your skin overly dry and tight. Furthermore, since soaps by their very nature are designed to be lathered onto your skin and then immediately washed off, any potentially valuable active antiacne ingredients that may be incorporated into them have insufficient contact time with your skin to be beneficial.

Keeping your face moist and supple enough to tolerate the use of real antiacne medications is a key point to remember. As you learned in the previous chapter, most currently available acne medications have the unfortunate side effect of leaving your skin slightly dry. Combined with the use of acne medications, superscrubbing can make you excessively and uncomfortably dry, particularly during the harsher and drier autumn and winter seasons. Even worse, the combination of excessively dry skin and persistent, active acne can be painful. In addition, if you have dark skin, dryness can leave your skin whitish and flaky-looking.

Drying out your skin by too harsh or too frequent cleansing can also initiate a vicious circle. People with overly washed skin often attempt to treat their dryness by applying heavy, oily moisturizing lotions and cosmetics after washing. Many of these products worsen acne by clogging pores and causing more breakouts. These flare-ups are, in turn, frequently met by still more vigorous washing; the cycle continues unless the excessive washing is stopped and replaced by gentle cleansing.

Rule #3: When selecting cosmetics, choose oil-free moisturizers, water-based or gel foundation makeups, and powder or gel blushes. In general, if you follow these guidelines, it matters little which brands you choose. Many American cosmetic houses test their products to be sure that they are noncomedogenic (non-acne-producing).

Rule #4: Avoid using astringents. Astringents are alcohol- or acetone-containing lotions that are supposed to dissolve excess skin oils and surface dirt and leave your skin feeling fresher and tighter. Unfortunately, overuse of astringents can result in dryness and flakiness. If you do choose to use astringents, use them judiciously. You may find them especially useful at times when you perspire heavily, such as following strenuous exercise or during extremely hot, humid weather (Table 4.2).

In general, regular soap-and-water cleansing is an effective way to manage oily skin. If you find that the oils reappear soon after cleaning, try blotting your skin periodically with a soft facial tissue to remove the excess oil. If you find simple blotting insufficient to control oiliness, you may try swabbing your face periodically with an individually packaged alcohol towelette (the kind your doctor uses to clean your skin before an injection). Alcohol towelettes are sterile and convenient to carry in your pocket or purse for use during the day as needed. If you prefer, you may also use plain witch hazel for this purpose or the commercial astringent **Seba-Nil** lotion.

Rule #5: Avoid using abrasive scrub brushes, polyester sponges, or washcloths to clean your skin. Like strong soaps or astringents, they simply contribute to dryness and irritation while providing little real benefit. Moreover, stretching the skin with these items can rupture whiteheads under the surface, further aggravating your condition.

Rule #6: Don't pick, squeeze, or scratch your pimples or whiteheads. Many parents make a crusade of this rule with their children. The temptation to "pop" your pimple will be great, but don't give in. Squeezing your pimples will often cause unsightly stains on your skin, which may persist for many weeks. Even worse, squeezing may cause permanent scarring. Finally, squeezing can break the skin and allow a secondary bacterial infection to occur.

NONPRESCRIPTION ANTIACNE MEDICATIONS

Most nonprescription (so-called over-the-counter) acne medications intended for home self-treatment consist of the following four ingredients found either alone or in combination: sulfur, resorcinol, salicylic acid, and benzoyl peroxide (Table 4.2). Over-the-counter medications, like the prescription medications that are discussed later in this chapter, are usually formulated as creams, lotions, gels, and masks.

Sulfur/Resorcinol

Sulfur alone, or combinations of sulfur and resorcinol, have been used for many years for both their skin-peeling (*keratolytic*) and antibacterial properties. These ingredients function best to speed the healing of pimples that are already present, rather than prevent the for-

TABLE 4.2
**SOME NONPRESCRIPTION
ACNE MEDICATIONS**

Astringents (alcohol swabs, witch hazel,
    Seba-Nil)
Sulfur/Resorcinol (Rezamid, Clearasil's
    Adult Care)
Salicylic Acid (Saligel, Stri-Dex Medicated
    Pads, Keralyt gel)
Benzoyl peroxide gels (Clear by Design,
    Fostex BPO 5 or 10)

mation of new ones. A number of sulfur/resorcinol-containing products are available as flesh-tinted lotions so that they may also be used as cover-ups for hiding blemishes. Almost always unwilling to use girls' makeups to cover blemishes, boys often find flesh-tinted acne medications to be especially useful products. Color blenders are provided with many of these products so that you can try to match them to your natural skin color.

For best results, first apply a small amount of the lotion directly over the blemish to be covered. Next, "feather" the edges of the medication to make it blend more naturally and gradually with the surrounding normal skin.

Unfortunately, even when great care is taken to produce a satisfactory color match, flesh-tinted lotions do not always precisely match your natural skin color. Furthermore, blacks and darker-skinned whites often complain of a whitish flakiness on their skin when these medications dry. Nevertheless, many people benefit from them.

Vlemasque is a sulfur-containing mask that is intended to be applied to your skin as a thick paste, left on for only twenty minutes, and then washed off.

Vlemasque is especially useful in treatment of moderately severe or severe forms of inflammatory acne.

You don't need to keep the medication on overnight, as you would most other antiacne medications. Some people even claim to find the mask soothing to their skin.

Salicylic Acid

Salicylic acid, another form of peeling agent, is particularly effective for treating blackheads. It appears to loosen and soften thick, clogged pores. Like sulfur and resorcinol, however, salicylic acid does little to prevent the development of new acne blemishes. Salicylic acid preparations are usually alcohol-based medications. The alcohol base provides the additional benefit of removing oil. Individuals with oily skin may find that these products leave their skin feeling cleaner and fresher.

Benzoyl Peroxide

Benzoyl peroxide is probably the single-most effective antiacne medication available without a prescription. It is available in creams, lotions, or gels in concentrations ranging from 2.5 percent to 10 percent. Unlike the other medications already mentioned, benzoyl peroxide is both effective in preventing the development of new blemishes and clearing up those already present.

It is believed to work in several ways. It unplugs pores by acting as a mild peeling agent on the inside of the hair follicles. It also penetrates the hair follicles, where it kills the bacteria capable of breaking down oil and debris buildup into potentially irritating, acne-producing fatty acids.

In general, benzoyl peroxide gels are believed to be more effective than benzoyl peroxide creams or lotions. Interestingly, recent studies indicate that the 5 percent and 10 percent concentrations aren't any more effective than the 2.5 percent concentration for controlling acne. Moreover, for most people, except those with the oiliest complexions, the higher concentration benzoyl peroxide products can be excessively chapping and irritating.

When applying any of these medications, you should avoid the sensitive areas near your eyes and lips; these areas tend to become easily irritated.

The majority of benzoyl peroxide gels currently available require a doctor's prescription. **Clear by Design,** however, is a nonprescription 2.5 percent benzoyl peroxide gel. **Fostex BPO,** which is available in both 5 percent and 10 percent concentrations, is another nonprescription gel.

Neutrogena's Acne Mask is a unique 5 percent benzoyl peroxide preparation. Like Vlemasque, it is designed to be applied as a thick paste mask, left on for twenty minutes, then washed off. The short duration of application seems to make dryness and irritation less of a problem. Once again, you don't need to sleep with the medication on.

A few final notes on self-treatment. No one product is right for everybody's skin. If you experience burning, itching, redness, or swelling after using any medication, you should immediately discontinue its use and let your skin rest for a day or two. If you continue to experience symptoms for more than a couple of days, you should seek medical attention. Always bear in mind that acne is a potentially scarring condition. This applies particularly to moderately severe or severe cases of acne that have been allowed to go untreated or have been improperly treated. Therefore, if you observe no improvement in your condition, or only minimal improvement, after three to four weeks of self-treatment, you should consult a dermatologist.

MEDICAL TREATMENT FOR ACNE

Although it is true that no cure has as yet been discovered for acne, you no longer need to live with pimples. You don't have to manage as best as you can until you outgrow the problem. During the past ten to fifteen years, active research into the causes and control of acne has led to the development of a wide variety of effective oral and topical prescription drugs. These

TABLE 4.3
MEDICAL TREATMENTS FOR ACNE

Benzoyl peroxide gels (water-, acetone-, or alcohol-based)

Retin-A (cream, lotion, or gel)

Oral antibiotics (tetracycline, minocycline, erythromycin)

Topical antibiotics (clindamycin, erythromycin, tetracycline)

Accutane

Acne surgery (comedone extraction; incision and drainage)

Therapeutic injections

include a wide variety of benzoyl peroxide gels, Retin-A, topical and oral antibiotics, and Accutane (Table 4.3). Even if you have an inherited tendency to have acne breakouts, these newer remedies can do much to make you look and feel as though you don't.

Several years ago, a study was performed to determine some of the more common misconceptions that patients have about acne and its treatments. Interestingly, nearly 40 percent of those studied had the unrealistic expectation that their acne would magically disappear within at most a month after medical therapy was begun. Unhappily, this is not yet the case. In fact, most topical medications that are prescribed by dermatologists do not even begin to work until about one week after they are started; furthermore, their maximal effects are not usually seen until about three to four weeks following the start of therapy. Contrary to popular belief, oral medications usually do not begin to work until about two to three weeks following the beginning of therapy, and their maximal effects may not be seen until six to eight weeks have elapsed. To be realistic, and to prevent yourself from experiencing needless upset and frustration, do not expect to see satisfactory improvement in your condition until between two and three *months* after you start proper medical therapy.

If permanent acne scarring has already occurred, your dermatologist can perform a number of cosmetic procedures to improve your appearance. For example, injections of collagen may be used to plump up depressed pockmark scars. Dermabrasion to "sand" scars down and make them less noticeable, can also be performed. These and other procedures are discussed in Chapter 11. Now let us look at the commonly prescribed antiacne medications.

Benzoyl Peroxides

Prescription benzoyl peroxide preparations are invariably gel formulations rather than creams or lotions. Gels may be water-based, alcohol-based, or acetone-based. Alcohol-based gels are usually the most drying and water-based the least. Your dermatologist will be able to choose the best preparation for your individual needs. Some of the more commonly prescribed products are: **Benzagel-5, Benzagel-10, Panoxyl 5** gel and **Panoxyl 10** gel (alcohol-based); **Persagel 5** gel and **Persagel 10** gel (acetone-based); and **Panoxyl Aq 2½** gel, **Panoxyl Aq 5** gel, and **Panoxyl Aq 10** gel (water-based). As mentioned earlier, it is best to start on a 2½ percent water-based benzoyl peroxide gel because these are generally the least irritating.

Retin-A

Retin-A (vitamin A acid, tretinoin), which is available in gel, liquid, or cream forms, is believed by many to be one of the most effective topical antiacne medications yet developed. As you already know, the plugging of your pores is the most important first step in the formation of pimples. Retin-A can reverse this process by making the plugged cells less sticky and by speeding the turnover of new cells within the lining of the pores. Improvement is usually seen between three to six weeks after starting therapy. Many people experience a temporary worsening of their condition about two weeks after starting. You should keep this in mind so that you don't become discouraged during the early stages of treatment. Retin-A has a tendency to be quite drying. To minimize this tendency, it should be used very sparingly and applied no less than twenty (preferably thirty) minutes following a face wash.

Oral Antibiotics

Although acne is not an infection, the bacterial organism *Propionobacterium acnes,* as you learned in Chapter 3, is nevertheless believed to play an important role in acne development. These bacteria are responsible for breaking down and converting the oils and debris trapped within clogged pores into irritating, acne-causing fatty acids. Both oral and topical antibiotics effectively suppress these bacteria.

Antibiotics are a mainstay of acne therapy. At one time, only oral antibiotics were available. Tetracycline has been a favorite for over thirty years. Erythromycin and minocycline are two other frequently prescribed oral antibiotics. However, since the introduction of topical antibiotics, oral antibiotics are now more frequently reserved for treating the most severe forms of acne.

When used to treat infections, oral antibiotics usually begin to work in a matter of hours. In treating acne, however, oral antibiotics usually do not bring about improvement for about three weeks.

Fortunately, the three oral antibiotics most commonly prescribed—tetracycline, erythromycin, and minocycline—have proven themselves generally safe even for long-term use. Minor, and often temporary, side effects include upset stomach, diarrhea, headache, and vaginal yeast infections. Your doctor is best able to choose the right oral antibiotic for your condition and may even switch you from one to the other, depending upon your response to treatment. Some of the more common brands of oral antibiotics prescribed include **Achromycin** (tetracycline), **Erythrocin, EES-400,** and **Eryc** capsules (erythromycin), and **Minocin** (minocycline).

Topical Antibiotics

One major disadvantage of taking antibiotics orally is that in order to treat acne on the face or chest, your whole system has to be unnecessarily exposed to the effects of the antibiotics. Topical antibiotics were developed to answer the need for antibiotics that work only where they are needed. Today, many patients who once would have required oral antibiotics may be treated with topical antibiotics. For more severe cases, however, your dermatologist may prescribe both a topical and an oral antibiotic.

Topical antibiotics are available as lotions, creams, or ointments. Lotions, which are usually alcohol-based, tend to be more drying and are usually reserved for patients with oilier skin. Creams and ointments, because they are moisturizing, are particularly useful for individuals with dry skin or for use during cold, chapping winter weather. Clindamycin, erythromycin, and tetracycline are three of the most commonly prescribed topical antibiotics. Your dermatologist may have the pharmacist tailor a topical antibiotic specifically for your needs or he or she may prescribe one of a variety of commercially available prescription preparations. Effective commercial preparations include **Cleocin-T** (clindamycin), **Staticin** lotion (1½ percent erythromycin), **T-Stat** and **Erymax** lotions (2 percent erythromycin), **Topicycline** lotion (tetracycline), **Meclan** cream (tetracycline derivative), and **Akne-mycin** ointment (2 percent erythromycin).

Erycette lotion is a recently introduced topical erythromycin. Individually prepackaged in sterile foil packets, Erycette consists of erythromycin-saturated towelettes. Many people like the convenience of this product, although it is more expensive.

Accutane (isotretinoin) is a potent oral vitamin A derivative. This drug may represent the single most significant advance to date in the treatment of severe, scarring cystic acne (Grade IV) of the face, chest, and back. Accutane has been shown to suppress oil-gland secretions, an effect that may last months after the drug has been discontinued. For many patients with severe, disfiguring cystic acne, for whom no other treatments have worked, Accutane has resulted in complete and long-lasting clearing of the skin.

Unfortunately, Accutane is not right for everyone. It has been associated with a number of side effects. These most commonly include extremely dry skin and severely chapped lips. Other common side effects include occasional nosebleeds, gum soreness, body aches and pains, itching, peeling of the palms and soles, increased sensitivity to the sun, and increased sensitivity to contact lenses. Most of these problems clear up once therapy is discontinued. More serious side effects include abnormal bone changes in the spine, blurred vision, hair loss, and elevated blood lipid (fat) levels. Most of these side effects also disappear once Accutane therapy is discontinued. In the case of bone changes, however, the effects may be permanent. Dermatologists are in the best position to determine which individuals will most profit from Accutane therapy. People taking the drug require frequent follow-up visits to their doctor and periodic blood tests to both monitor their progress and look for adverse reactions.

Although acne may actually worsen during the first few weeks of Accutane therapy, significant improvement can usually be seen by the tenth to twelfth week. A full course of therapy usually lasts between sixteen and twenty weeks. If necessary, a second course of therapy may be given two months later.

Other Kinds of Acne Treatments

Often, in addition to the use of oral or topical agents, your dermatologist will perform a "cleansing" of your skin. Acne surgery is the technical name for the removal of blackheads and whiteheads and the opening and draining of acne cysts. Instead of having to wait several weeks to first observe the benefits of topical or oral antiacne remedies, the effects of acne surgery are more immediate.

Comedo extraction, or having your blackheads and whiteheads removed, can often make you look better and feel better about yourself almost immediately. Even more importantly, by removing whiteheads before they can evolve into pimples and cysts, the likelihood of future breakouts is decreased. For this reason, many dermatologists maintain that acne surgery is one of the single most important treatments for acne.

Incision and drainage, or the opening up and draining of inflamed cysts and abscesses, is another important type of acne surgery. If performed early, before too much damage has occurred, incision and drainage procedures can speed healing and reduce the risk of scarring. If done correctly, both types of acne surgery— comedo extraction and incision and drainage—should cause only minimal discomfort and result in no scarring.

Cystic lesions and abscesses may also be treated by the use of therapeutic (intralesional) injections. Therapeutic injections consist of instilling a small amount of an anti-inflammatory medication directly into deep cysts or abscesses in order to reduce inflammation and possible scar formation. Such injections can be used alone or in combination with incision and drainage, depending upon the specific circumstances. Since the medication is injected exactly where it is most needed, little is required and almost none is absorbed into the rest of the body. Following injection, cysts and abscesses usually go down within twelve to forty-eight hours. As a rule, if you develop acne cysts or abscesses, you should see your dermatologist as soon as possible. The longer that you permit large, inflamed cysts to remain before seeking proper treatment, the greater your risk of developing permanent scars.

5

Common Skin Rashes
and Infections

Many different kinds of rashes can affect your skin. Doctors sometimes refer to rashes as *eruptions*. Some eruptions are caused by infectious germs, such as bacteria, fungi (sing., *fungus*), or viruses. Other rashes are noninfectious in nature. Fortunately, most common rashes are not serious but can become quite unsightly, annoying, and uncomfortable if left untreated. In Chapters 3 and 4, you learned about acne, which is one type of common noninfectious skin inflammation. In this chapter, you will learn about the causes, prevention, and treatments of a variety of other common rashes (Table 5.1).

COMMON
NONINFECTIOUS RASHES

Eczema (Dermatitis)
Eczema, or *dermatitis*, as most dermatologists prefer to call it, is a term used to cover a variety of skin conditions, many of which resemble each other closely both to the naked eye and under the microscope. As a rule, eczemas are very itchy and uncomfortable eruptions. Atopic,

contact, and seborrheic dermatitis are three of the more common types of eczema. Since they are not caused by germs, eczemas are *not* contagious.

In general, eczemas have three different stages, each with its own distinguishing features. These stages are referred to as the *acute, subacute,* and *chronic* stages. Depending upon the specific condition and circumstances, a patient with eczema may experience only one stage or pass through all three.

Acute eczema, the first stage, starts with some redness, swelling, and itching, then quickly progresses to the formation of blisters and oozing. Itching can be severe, but scratching and abrading the skin only intensify the itch and make infection more likely. However, contrary to popular belief and despite often profuse

---

TABLE 5.1 COMMON RASHES
AND INFECTIONS OF THE SKIN

NONINFECTIOUS RASHES	INFECTIOUS RASHES		
	Bacterial (pyodermas)	Fungal (ringworms)	Viral
Atopic Dermatitis	Impetigo	Tinea capitis	Herpes
Allergic Contact Dermatitis	Folliculitis	Tinea cruris	Molluscum
Irritant Contact Dermatitis	Furunculosis (boils)	Tinea pedis	Condyloma
Seborrhea and Seborrheic Dermatitis	Carbuncles (abscesses)	Tinea corporis	Veruccae (warts)
Keratosis Pilaris		Tinea versicolor (non-ringworm)	
Psoriasis			
Scabies			Parasite

oozing, eczemas are not contagious (except for those that have become secondarily infected with bacteria). Therefore, they cannot be spread to other parts of your body or to other people.

Subacute eczema, the second stage, is characterized by the presence of fewer blisters and less oozing. However, redness and scratch marks can be quite prominent.

Chronic eczema, the third stage, is characterized by dark, thick, and often cracked, leathery skin. Such changes represent the skin's reaction to persistent scratching and rubbing. At this stage, redness, blisters, and oozing are usually no longer present.

Atopic dermatitis is a very common eczema that affects about 3 percent of the U. S. population. It tends to occur in people whose families have tendencies toward eczema, asthma, hay fever, and hives. Although most people outgrow their eczema by their teen years, some, unfortunately, do not. In these individuals, the condition may persist throughout life. People with atopic dermatitis usually also suffer with excessively dry, sensitive skin.

Individuals with atopic dermatitis have periods of ups and downs. At one moment they may be completely free of their problem, and at the next, they may experience a flare-up. Flare-ups can be triggered by emotional upsets, physical stresses (such as colds, fevers, or sore throats), too much soap and water, or rapid shifts in the weather, especially in the winter when the air is dry. Foods seldom play a triggering role in atopic dermatitis, except in some young children, where the ingestion of citrus fruits, eggs, or milk may occasionally trigger flare-ups.

Although no cure is available for atopic dermatitis, once your doctor has made the diagnosis, a number of remedies may be prescribed to alleviate the symptoms. Topical corticosteroids (special prescription anti-inflammatory creams and lotions) have become the mainstays for treating severe eczema. Antihistamine (anti-itch and sedative) pills are also commonly prescribed to control an acute flare-up. Since infections may either trigger or complicate an attack of dermatitis, oral antibiotics are also often prescribed. Oral anti-inflammatory steroids are reserved for the most severe, difficult-to-control cases. Once under control, gentle soap-and-water cleansings, decreased bathing, and the daily, liberal use of moisturizers are strongly advised to reduce the chance of recurrence; moist and soft skin is less likely to develop flare-ups.

Contact dermatitis, as the name implies, is a rash resulting from the contact of an irritating substance with your skin. Two types of contact dermatitis may occur. One type is a true allergic reaction and is aptly called *allergic contact dermatitis.* The second type, which results from rubbing or other direct mechanical irritation, is called *irritant contact dermatitis.* Unlike other types of eczemas, neither allergic nor irritant contact eczemas are hereditary nor are they aggravated by emotional or physical stresses.

Some of the more common causes of allergic contact dermatitis include allergies to hair sprays, shampoos, hair dyes, jewelry, cosmetics, topical medications, and poison ivy. Sometimes, the location and shape of the allergic rash will give your dermatologist a clue to the substances that caused it. For example, contact allergy to a shoe leather dye would appear on the sides and tops of your feet, and poison ivy appears in streaks, where the branches or leaves of the plant brushed against the skin.

Interestingly, as a rule, it takes several encounters with an allergy-causing substance to develop an allergy to it. The first time you manifest an allergic contact eczema to a substance may actually be the second, hundredth, or thousandth time that you have actually come into contact with the particular offending substance. Put another way, it takes time and multiple experiences to develop an allergy to a particular material.

Irritant contact dermatitis, on the other hand, is *not* an allergic reaction. Instead, it results from either prolonged contact with a mildly irritating substance or brief contact with a highly irritating substance. Examples of substances that may result in the development of irritant eczema include harsh soaps and detergents, acids, alkalis, and solvents (such as turpentine). Unlike allergic dermatitis, an irritant reaction typically occurs upon the first exposure.

Medical treatment for contact dermatitis is nearly the same as that for atopic dermatitis. In the case of contact dermatitis, however, an "ounce of prevention is truly worth a pound of cure." Prevention of subsequent episodes of either allergic or irritant contact dermatitis consists, first and foremost, of avoiding contact with any known offending substances.

Seborrheic dermatitis is a common form of recurring eczema. Millions of people are affected by it at one time or another. Regions of the body having the greatest concentrations of sebaceous (oil) glands are most often affected. These include the face, scalp, central chest and back, armpits, navel, and groin.

Although the cause of seborrheic dermatitis remains unknown, heredity is believed to play some role. Often, seborrheic dermatitis worsens when you are under a great deal of emotional stress. It may also flare up during periods of physical stress, such as when you are suffering from colds, fevers, sore throats, or allergy attacks. Seborrheic dermatitis is *not* a contagious condition.

The signs and symptoms of seborrheic dermatitis can range from quite mild to severe. In its mildest form, seborrheic dermatitis is referred to simply as *seborrhea*, or plain dandruff. Seborrhea is characterized by itchiness and unsightly flaking. More severe forms of seborrheic dermatitis are characterized by larger patches of redness, flaking, and thick crusting.

Although no cure is yet available, most cases of seborrheic dermatitis can easily be controlled. Routine use of a commercial, nonprescription antidandruff shampoo is all that is ordinarily necessary to control mild cases of simple dandruff. Dandruff shampoos most often contain one or more of the following active ingredients: zinc pyrithione, sulfur, salicylic acid, or tars. **Sebulon, Sebulex, Ionil,** and **T-Gel** are examples of shampoos containing these active ingredients.

More severe cases of scalp and facial seborrheic dermatitis frequently require consultation with a dermatologist. Your doctor may prescribe a more potent shampoo, one containing 2 percent selenium sulfide, such as **Exsel** or **Selsun.** In addition, one of a wide variety of corticosteroid (anti-inflammatory) lotions or gels may be required. Even the most severe cases of seborrheic dermatitis can be controlled with the combined use of these shampoos and prescription medications. Once satisfactory control is achieved, you can maintain a dandruff-free scalp with routine use of one of the commercial antidandruff shampoos. For maintaining clear facial skin, your doctor may prescribe the occasional use of one of the milder topical corticosteroids.

Keratosis Pilaris
("Prickly hair follicles")

Keratosis pilaris is a condition that is so commonly seen that it can almost be considered a variant of normal skin. It occurs mostly during the teen years. Keratosis pilaris appears as numerous reddish, rough, spiny little bumps located at the openings of the pores. These bumps are most often observed on the outer arms and outer thighs. They are sometimes confused with pimples. Affected areas of skin look and feel like coarse sandpaper. Keratosis pilaris is more widespread in patients who also have atopic dermatitis. In the majority of patients, keratosis pilaris improves and eventually disappears entirely somewhere in their twenties or thirties.

Since keratosis pilaris by itself is a perfectly harmless condition, no treatment is usually necessary. Reassurance that their condition is harmless and will eventually disappear is ordinarily all that most people with this condition need. However, if the eruption becomes extensive, it can pose significant cosmetic and psychological problems. In that case, your doctor can set up a program for you, consisting of daily buffing with an abrasive sponge and the use of high-potency moisturizers, such as **Lac-Hydrin** lotion. On occasion, a mild topical anti-inflammatory corticosteroid may also be required.

Psoriasis

Psoriasis is a chronic condition that affects about 5 million Americans and nearly 3 percent of the world's population. Heredity appears to play an important role. For those having a hereditary predisposition to psoriasis, increased nervous tension and physical stresses may aggravate the condition or trigger a flare-up. Other aggravating factors include overly dry skin, sunburn, sore throats, and cuts or scrapes of the skin. Psoriasis is *not* a contagious condition.

In psoriasis, skin cells are produced at a rate about 2 to 7 times more quickly than in normal skin (Fig. 5.1). Instead of being shed rapidly, however, the cells in psoriasis typically stick together to form thick, whitish scaly patches. Flaking from psoriasis of the scalp may occasionally be confused with simple dandruff, although the flaking and irritation of psoriasis is generally more severe and resistant to commercial antidandruff shampoos.

Psoriasis may affect any area of the skin, including the scalp and nails. Although sometimes causing itching, in most cases psoriasis causes few physical symptoms. When large areas of the body are involved, psoriasis can pose significant cosmetic and psychological problems.

Although active research continues for a cure for psoriasis, satisfactory therapies are currently available. All but the mildest cases should be under the close supervision of a dermatologist experienced in treating psoriasis. Therapy consists of slowing down the abnormally rapid skin cell growth rate, alleviating symptoms if present, and keeping the skin moist.

Effective psoriasis therapies include the use of prescription topical anti-inflammatory corticosteroid creams,

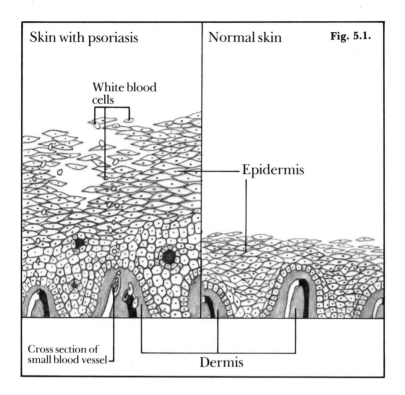

| Skin with psoriasis | Normal skin | **Fig. 5.1.** |

White blood cells

Epidermis

Cross section of small blood vessel

Dermis

Psoriasis Under the Microscope

lotions, and ointments, therapeutic injections of triam-
cinolone for particularly stubborn patches, and antidandruff shampoos for scalp psoriasis. Each of these types
of therapy has already been covered in other sections.

Other treatments for psoriasis include the use of
coal tar or anthralin (petroleum derivatives) in cream,
lotion, or paste forms. Tars and anthralins are used for
their anti-inflammatory properties and for their abilities
to slow down the rate of skin cell production. Sunlight
or artificial ultraviolet light exposure (using UVB),
either alone or in combination with the application of
skin moisturizers, coal tar derivatives, or anthralin, has

also been found effective, particularly for more resistent or widespread cases of psoriasis.

PUVA (*p*soralen plus *u*ltra*v*iolet light *A*) therapy is a relatively new, and highly effective, form of ultraviolet light psoriasis treatment. Psoralens are chemicals that make psoriasis patients sensitive to the benefits of UVA light. Encouraging results have thus far been seen. in clearing patients with extensive psoriasis and keeping them clear.

Finally, a new oral vitamin A derivative, **Tegason** (etretinate), a relative of Accutane, which has been in use in Europe for several years, has just received FDA approval for use in the United States. It has shown tremendous promise in the management of severe forms of psoriasis, either alone or in combination with PUVA treatment. All other therapies must be administered under close medical supervision. Happily, psoriasis sufferers today have much reason for optimism.

COMMON INFECTIOUS RASHES

Ringworm

"Ringworm" is the common, and probably the most frequently used, name for contagious infections of the skin caused by yeastlike germs called *fungi*. These infections have nothing to do with worms, however. Typically, the infections appear as reddish, scaly rings, hence the name. Fungal infections frequently also cause blistering, cracking, and dry scaling of the skin. Fungal involvement of the fingernails and toenails can lead to thickened, yellow, distorted, crumbling, and loose nails. Itching and burning are the most common symptoms of ringworm. Doctors refer to ringworm infections as *tineas*; ringworm of the feet, or "athlete's foot," is referred to as *tinea pedis*; ringworm of the groin, or "jock itch," is known as *tinea cruris*; ringworm of the scalp is called *tinea capitis;* and ringworm of the entire body is named *tinea corporis*.

A dermatologist's help is often needed to diagnose ringworm infections, as their appearance often mimics eczemas or psoriasis. In addition to examining the affected skin, your doctor may need to examine skin scrapings under the microscope and take cultures to establish the diagnosis.

Fortunately, most tineas are caused by only a few different kinds of related fungi and all may be treated in the same manner. Antifungal creams and lotions are usually all that are necessary to eliminate most fungal infections of the skin. Several effective OTC products include **Monostat, Tinactin**, and **Desenex**. For scalp and nail infections, however, an oral antifungal antibiotic, griseofulvin, is frequently required as well. Fingernail infections may take six to twelve months to cure and toenail infections twelve to eighteen months.

Antifungal treatment must be continued until all fungi have been eradicated. In the course of treatment, it is not enough for your skin just to feel better. It is not even enough for the affected areas to look completely clear. In order to minimize the chance of the infection returning, your doctor will probably repeat the fungal culture to ensure that no microscopic fungal organisms remain on your skin. Treatment can be discontinued once a repeat fungal culture demonstrates no organisms.

Simple measures can help decrease the chance of spreading or contracting ringworm infections. To prevent ringworm of the scalp, you should avoid sharing combs, brushes, hats, or headgear with anyone else. Because ringworm can also be spread from pets, you should be sure to have any skin or fur problems in pets immediately examined by a veterinarian. Since fungi require moisture, warmth, and darkness to spread, to prevent athlete's foot keep your feet dry and clean. Be sure to dry your feet thoroughly after bathing or exercising. Remove any debris that accumulates between your toes. Avoid using moisture-trapping heavy woolen socks; instead, use cotton socks. Wear sandals during warm weather and lightly dust your feet, shoes, and socks daily with an antifungal dusting powder, such as **Zeasorb-AF**, Desenex, or Tinactin.

Tinea versicolor

Tinea versicolor is another type of common fungal infection. It is unrelated to ringworm infections, although it is sometimes confused with them. Tinea versicolor is seen worldwide and accounts for about 5 percent of all fungal infections. This fungus most commonly involves the neck, trunk, and arms; the face, however, is rarely involved. Tinea versicolor seldom causes any symptoms, but if it becomes widespread, it can be quite noticeable and embarrassing, especially during the sunny summer months. Because patches of tinea versicolor frequently become more apparent during the summer, some patients *mistakenly* attribute them to sun exposure and call them "sunspots."

Spots of tinea versicolor are oval, show fine scales, and may be variously colored from white to pink or brown (hence, the name *versi*color). In many cases your doctor can confirm the diagnosis by examining some of the fungus-containing scales under the microscope. He or she may also look for the fungus by shining a special ultraviolet light on your skin, called a Wood's light. Tinea versicolor will often exhibit an orange-gold color when exposed to this form of light.

Treating tinea versicolor consists of the application of antifungal creams, such as those used to treat ringworm, or by the application of a selenium sulfide shampoo (**Excel** or **Selsun**). A more potent oral medication, ketoconazole (**Nizoral**), is occasionally required to treat more resistent or recurrent cases. This medication remains a measure of last resort because of its potential side effects. Finally, since the tinea versicolor fungus ordinarily interferes with normal suntanning, even after you are cured, it may take months for your skin's color to even out and return to normal.

COMMON BACTERIAL INFECTIONS OF THE SKIN (PYODERMAS)

Skin infections, or *pyodermas*, are caused by a variety of bacteria (germs). Staphylococcus and streptococcus, frequently referred to as staph and strep for short, are the two kinds of bacteria responsible for the majority of skin infections.

If a bacterial infection is limited to the uppermost layers of your skin, it is referred to as *impetigo* (pronounced im-puh-TIE-go). Patches of impetigo typically manifest themselves as extremely itchy, reddish, oozing patches covered by honey-colored crusts. Impetigo is highly contagious.

If an infection is located high up near the top of a hair follicle (pore), it is referred to as *folliculitis*. Folliculitis, which is often itchy, resembles small pustules of acne. Several years ago, during the height of the tight jeans and disco craze, many cases of folliculitis of the buttocks were observed, owing to the constant rubbing of the jeans against the follicles on the buttocks. The condition became so common that dermatologist's nicknamed it "disco dermatitis."

If the bacteria spread more deeply into the hair follicle, the resulting infection is known as *furunculosis* (boils). Warm, red, and tender boils may resemble ordinary pimples. Should the infection continue to spread to areas outside the hair follicles, the resulting infections are called *carbuncles*. Carbuncles, which are red, hot, painful abscesses filled with pus, debris, dead skin cells, and bacteria, are larger and deeper than boils.

Curing bacterial infections generally requires the use of both topical and oral antibiotics. Your doctor may suggest that you apply warm-water compresses several times daily or soak in a warm tub. In addition, he or she will probably recommend the use of nonprescription topical antibiotic ointments, such as **Polysporin** or **Bacitracin.**

Deeper carbuncles will usually require incision and drainage, under local anesthesia. At no time should you attempt to squeeze boils or carbuncles. If you do, you risk making the infection worse. You also risk introducing bacteria into your bloodstream and causing a serious condition called *septicemia* ("blood poisoning").

VIRAL INFECTIONS
OF THE SKIN

Herpes, molluscum contagiosum, condyloma acuminatum (venereal warts), and verrucae (warts) are currently the most common infections of the skin. Although herpes, molluscum, and venereal warts may be spread by nonsexual means, the transmission of these conditions today so commonly occurs through sexual contact that they are usually included in the category of sexually transmitted diseases.

The medical name for warts is *verrucae*. Warts are caused by a virus called the human papillomavirus. More than forty different types of closely related human papillomaviruses are known to exist. Warts are usually named by either how they look or where they grow. For example, *verruca plana*, or the flat wart, gets its name because of its smooth, flat top; *verruca plantaris*, or plantar wart, gets its name because it grows on the bottom of the foot. (Plantar refers to the sole of the foot and has nothing to do with the word plant*er*, as some people mistakenly believe.)

Prior trauma to the skin plays an important role in the development of warts. This is believed to be the reason why your hands and feet, areas subjected to frequent injury, are the most common locations affected by them. Although in most cases unsightly and the cause of considerable embarrassment, warts are usually painless. In certain locations, however, such as the feet, they can cause extreme discomfort and even disability.

Each type of wart has distinguishing features. Common warts are flesh-colored, rough-surfaced bumps. Flat warts are smooth-surfaced and flat-topped, and plantar warts are flat, heavily callused areas on the bottom of the feet. All warts contain little black specks, which represent tiny wart blood vessels.

Wart infections can progress in one of several ways. Warts that you have now may persist in their current form unchanged for many years. Or they may spread. Or they may disappear spontaneously as your body's immune system succeeds in fighting them off. The fact that warts can spontaneously disappear probably accounts for the many "successes" of folk remedies. Some of these remedies to "witch away" warts included rubbing them with stones then burying the stones, rubbing them with potatoes, ear wax, and so on.

Today, a variety of medications and procedures are available for ridding you of unsightly or painful warts. Your dermatologist may recommend the home use of medications containing strong acids, such as salicylic and lactic acid (**Tiflex, Occlusal,** and **Viranol).** Unfortunately, the use of these acids is not uniformly successful. Even when effective, acids may take six to twelve weeks to work. Caustic substances such as cantharadin or trichloroacetic acid, or freezing solutions such as liquid nitrogen, are also sometimes recommended. Often, more than one treatment session is required. Electrocautery, or the use of a heat-producing electric current to destroy wart tissue, is another method. It is quick and offers the least chance for recurrence. Performed under local anesthesia, the entire procedure takes about five minutes and is virtually painless.

SCABIES

Scabies is a highly contagious skin disease caused by a nearly invisible parasitic bug, *Sarcoptes scabiei,* the "itch mite." The tiny organism burrows into the skin to cause irritation and allergy. Scabies is acquired largely through close physical contact, but may also be spread through contaminated clothing, linens, and towels. There is a four- to six-week incubation period between the time of exposure and the outbreak of the rash.

Scabies typically affects the webbed spaces between the fingers and toes, the back of the hands, the wrists, elbows, armpits, breasts, and beltline, and the genital area and buttocks; the face is typically spared. In general, the rash is extremely itchy, particularly at night, and mite burrows appear as grayish-white, threadlike streaks, tiny blisters, and scratched pimplelike bumps.

Unfortunately, infestation with scabies does not confer any permanent immunity against future attacks. In fact, if you have had scabies before, subsequent attacks are more severe and generally occur after shorter incubation periods. Daily shampooing, good personal grooming habits, and not sharing clothing, bedding, or towels with friends are good methods for preventing scabies infestations. Above all, close contact with anyone complaining of a rash that is especially itchy at night should be avoided until a dermatologist has been consulted.

Cure is available. **Kwell** and **Scabene** lotions, which contain the potent pesticide lindane, are most often prescribed for this condition. The lotion is applied at bedtime to all the affected areas and rinsed off in the morning. All intimate apparel should be either hot-water laundered or dry-cleaned.

6

Hair Care

Most people would agree that having a thick, healthy looking head of hair is vital for a good appearance. Millions of dollars are spent each year by consumers looking for products to shampoo "life" into their hair, condition it, remove scales and tangles, add body, and counteract dryness and "flyaway" hair. Millions more are spent to change its color, or straighten or curl it. With so many hair-care products to choose from and so much hype about the supposed benefits of these products, selecting the right products for proper hair and scalp care can be very confusing.

BASIC FACTS ABOUT
NORMAL HAIR

The first myth about your hair that must be debunked is that it is "alive." Nobody's hair is alive. Hair, like the topmost layer of your skin, is composed of the nonliving fibrous protein substance keratin. The truly living and reproducing region of each hair, the so-called *root,* lies buried deep below the scalp surface, at the base of each hair follicle (Fig. 6.1). The living cells within the hair

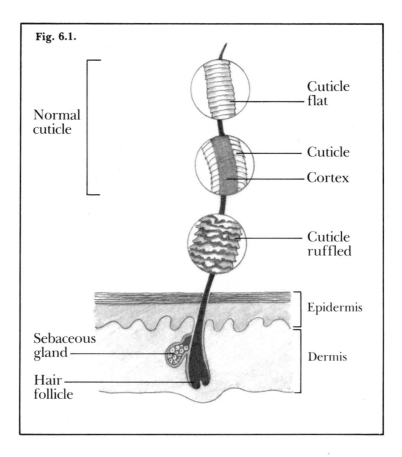

Hair Follicle and Hair Shaft

root produce the nonliving fibrous strands that we call hair.

Hair strands are composed of two main layers. The outer layer is called the *cuticle.* Arranged in overlapping layers, the cuticle protects the cortex from fraying and splitting. The inner layer, which is called the *cortex,* provides support for the hairs. Since hair fibers are no more alive than clothing fibers, contrary to what some product manufacturers would like you to believe, no hair-care product can "nourish," "feed," or "rejuvenate" your hair or make it "come alive."

The number of hairs that you have and their color, type, texture, length, and thickness are inherited traits. On an average, most people with a full head of hair possess a total of about 100,000 hairs. Redheads have fewer but thicker hairs—approximately 80,000. On the other hand, blondes have a greater number but thinner hairs—approximately 120,000 hairs. Brunettes fall somewhere in between, both in the number and thickness of individual hairs. You may be surprised to learn that a healthy person with a normal head of hair loses between fifty and a hundred hairs each day. As a rule, these hairs are replaced by an equal number of newly produced hairs.

Hair growth proceeds in phases—a growing phase, a resting phase, and a falling-out phase. Growth tends to be faster in the summer than in the winter, but on an average, hairs grow approximately half an inch (1.25 cm) each month. Individual hairs usually grow for about three to ten years before falling out and being replaced.

Whether you have curly, wavy, or straight hair is determined largely by two types of chemical bonds present within the proteins of each hair, hydrogen bonds and sulfur bonds. Hydrogen bonds are very weak bonds. Simply wetting your hair with water is enough to temporarily weaken them. This is why wet hair is easier to style. Sulfur bonds are strong bonds. Therefore, for more lasting hair styling, such as permanent waves or hair straightening, the sulfur bonds must be weakened by chemical reactions.

GENERAL TIPS ON HAIR CARE

Shampoo your hair as often as you need, daily if necessary, to control oiliness or flaking. Daily shampooing will not damage your hair nor cause hair loss. If you have dry hair, shampoo less often and use a conditioner (see below).

After shampooing, lightly *pat* your hair and scalp

dry. Do not vigorously towel dry them. Damp hair should first be combed with a wide-tooth comb and only later brushed, after your hair has dried thoroughly. Daily brushing can help to remove scales, dirt, and tangles and add luster to your hair. Brush only your hair, *not the scalp*. Natural tapered bristle brushes (frequently made from boar's hairs), rather than blunt synthetic bristle brushes (usually nylon), are less likely to scratch your scalp. Ball-tipped synthetic bristles, which have become very popular these days, are also gentle to the scalp.

Despite what you may have heard, blow-drying your hair can be safe—if you follow a few simple rules. Hold the blow-dryer no closer than 6 to 12 inches (15 to 30 cm) from your hair. Use cooler and slower air flow settings and do *not* overdry your hair. Leave your hair slightly damp.

Finally, avoid hairstyles that place a great deal of pull on your hair and scalp, such as ponytails, tight braids, and "cornrows." Prolonged tension on hairs, particularly dyed or bleached hair, can result in breakage. Even worse, temporary—and occasionally permanent—hair loss can result from the repeated, long-term use of tight-pulling styles or the overuse of brush rollers (see traction alopecia, below).

SHAMPOOS

The primary job of a shampoo is simply to cleanse your hair of dirt and excess oils. Soaps or detergents are the main ingredients in any shampoo. Years ago, people shampooed their hair with plain bar toilet soap. Toilet soaps cleaned well and were inexpensive. Even today, some people still use bar soap for shampooing.

However, for the most part, soaps are overdrying to the hair and can leave it dull and lifeless-looking. For that reason, most people now prefer commercial shampoos for cleaning their hair and scalp. In general, commercial shampoos leave your hair looking, feeling, and smelling better. The overwhelming majority of today's shampoos contain synthetic detergents and are considerably more expensive than plain bar soap.

A major advantage in using more expensive, synthetic detergent shampoos over plain bar soap is that, when used in hard water, they don't leave a scum deposit either on your hair or in the sink or tub. Hard water contains minerals, usually calcium and magnesium, which, as they settle, form scum deposits when mixed with plain soaps. Scum deposits make hair appear dull and lusterless. Synthetic detergents clean no better than plain soap. In general, detergent shampoos are quite similar in makeup to *mild* dishwashing liquids. In fact, if you wish, you could shampoo with a mild dishwashing liquid and save money.

Manufacturers frequently alter the basic shampoo formula to suit different purposes. Shampoos intended for oily or normal hair usually contain either greater amounts of one particular detergent or several strong detergents. On the other hand, "no more tears" shampoos for children contain the mildest detergents; they also lack other potentially irritating or eye-stinging ingredients, such as perfumes. Shampoos for dry hair often contain moisturizing conditioners.

Owing to their general alkalinity, most shampoos roughen the protective cuticle of the hair. This can result in dull, difficult-to-manage hair. As normal oil-gland secretions return to normal after shampooing, however, this ruffling effect *normally* disappears on its own in one to two days. To counter detergent alkalinity and to speed cuticle unruffling, so-called low-pH, non-alkaline, and pH-balanced shampoos have been formulated. These kinds of shampoos contain acids, such as citric or tartaric acids.

Formulated as creams, lotions, gels, or pastes, commercial shampoos may contain coloring, thickening, foaming, and lathering agents, as well as fragrances to improve their look, feel, and smell. Interestingly, a shampoo does *not* have to lather well to clean well. In the final analysis, since most products are about equally effective for cleaning your hair, your personal preferences for the look, feel, and smell of a shampoo and, of course, your budget will determine which brand you ultimately choose.

CONDITIONING SHAMPOOS, CREME RINSES, AND CONDITIONERS

Shampoos for naturally dry, bleached, or permed hair usually contain milder detergents, as well as conditioners. Conditioners are ingredients that moisturize hair, add body and gloss, and eliminate tangles and static. Shampoos containing both detergents and conditioners are referred to as conditioning shampoos. Creme rinses, or simply conditioners, are products made to be used as separate, after-shampoo, conditioning rinses. Conditioning shampoos and conditioners usually contain one or all of the following three types of ingredients: moisturizers, proteins, and quarternium compounds.

Moisturizing conditioners, commonly lanolin, balsam, or vegetable oils, are particularly useful for moisturizing hair after it has been "stripped" by routine shampooing. Moisturizers can also reduce static and "flyaway" hair. Protein conditioners, particularly those containing hydrolyzed animal proteins, bind *temporarily* to individual hair strands. They make hair appear shinier and fuller ("add body"). They can also *temporarily* bind split or frayed ends. Quarternium compounds are particularly effective for reducing static and improving combability. Finally, egg, lemon juice, and herbal additives, which you may also find in some conditioners, add little—except to the price of the conditioner.

If you require a conditioner, you would generally do better to use a separate creme rinse or conditioner *after* your regular shampoo, rather than a conditioning shampoo. Unquestionably more convenient, the idea of using all-in-one conditioning shampoos for both cleaning and conditioning your hair is attractive. Unfortunately, since the effects of detergent and conditioning ingredients often run counter to each other, using a separate shampoo and conditioner will generally prove more effective for most people.

MEDICATED SHAMPOOS

Medicated shampoos, as their name implies, are shampoos to which drugs have been added to prevent or treat a variety of scalp conditions. Medicated shampoos are particularly useful for controlling itching, dandruff, seborrheic dermatitis, and psoriasis (see Chapter 5). These shampoos may contain a variety of effective ingredients, such as zinc pyrithione, sulfur, salicylic acid, selenium sulfide, and tar derivatives. Zinc pyrithione and sulfur are used for their antiseptic properties, sulfur and salicylic acid for their peeling (descaling) abilities, and selenium sulfide and tars for their capacity to slow down the abnormal growth rate of skin cells in certain conditions.

Many medicated shampoos are available without prescription. For less severe scalp problems, you might try **Danex, Zincon,** or **Head and Shoulders** shampoos. For more severe conditions, **Sebulon, Sebulex, Selsun-Blue, X-Seb, Ionil-Plus,** or **T-Gel** shampoos are often effective.

In the beginning, you may need to use a medicated shampoo several times per week to achieve satisfactory control. Once control is achieved, however, you may find shampooing once or twice a week adequate to maintain control. For best results, you should leave the shampoo on your scalp for *at least* five minutes before rinsing. Of course, if you have any specific problems or questions, see your dermatologist.

HAIR COLORING

Three basic types of hair-coloring products are available: temporary, semipermanent, and permanent dyes. As their names suggest, these three types of dyes differ largely in how long the color lasts. In general, a temporary dye, also called a rinse, produces a color that lasts only until your next shampooing. A semipermanent dye may last through five or six shampoos, and a permanent dye remains permanently. The roots of your hair will, of course, grow out with your natural hair color.

In general, temporary dyes are relatively safe to use. They serve best to brighten and add highlights to hair. Temporary dyes cannot make darker shades lighter. They may occasionally rub off on your pillowcase and clothes. They can also run with heavy perspiration. Like temporary dyes, semipermanent dyes also primarily serve to brighten and highlight hair color. They, too, cannot make your hair lighter. Semipermanent coloration is sometimes used for color touch-ups in between permanent dye treatments.

Permanent dyes, also called oxidation dyes or tints, are the most frequently used of all three types of hair colorants. Permanent dyes are available for both home or professional salon use. These dyes are capable of producing hair colors many shades lighter than natural. To accomplish this, they require a developer (usually 6 percent hydrogen peroxide)—a bleach—to be mixed with the dye directly before use. Unfortunately, bleaching damages hair and makes it dry, brittle, fragile, and strawlike. Bleaching particularly damages the cuticle and therefore is not recommended.

HAIR-SETTING PREPARATIONS

Depending upon fashion changes, converting naturally straight hair to curly or curly hair to straight has been popular for several decades. A variety of commercial products are available for *temporarily* setting your hair in a particular style. These include hair sprays, setting lotions, hair fixatives, setting gels, and mousses. In general, these cosmetics work by weakening the hydrogen bonds in hair and by coating hairs with a transparent, semirigid gum or resin. Many also contain conditioners for moisturizing your hair and reducing static and tangles.

Temporary setting preparations are applied after the hair has been shampooed and set in rollers. The semirigid resin coating not only holds the set but serves to lock out moisture in order to hold the set longer. Setting preparations do not damage hair, although they are occasionally responsible for causing allergic reactions or irritations at the hairline.

ELECTRIC SETTING DEVICES

Electric rollers can be useful for giving a quick, temporary set. The heat generated by electric rollers breaks the weaker hydrogen bonds in hair, allowing the hair to be temporarily styled as desired. Overuse of electric rollers can be damaging, however, leaving your hair dry and brittle. Tinted or bleached hair can be particularly sensitive. In general, hot-mist (steam-heated) rollers are better than straight electric rollers because the mist serves to replenish some of the moisture lost by the heating process.

Electric curling irons can also be useful for quick styling. Like electric rollers, they work by weakening the hydrogen bonds within hair. Curling irons, however, tend to be hotter than electric rollers. Consequently, *extreme care* should be exercised when using them. Improper or excessive use of curling irons can result in dryness, brittleness, and burnt hair; burns of the scalp have also resulted.

PERMANENT WAVING

Permanent waving, or simply perming, is a process for changing straight hair to wavy or curly. Perming first involves breaking the strong sulfur bonds within hair. Once these bonds are broken, hair may be realigned to the desired degree of waviness or curliness. The process consists of placing the hair in rollers and then applying a bond-breaking chemical, which is allowed to remain in contact with the hair for about fifteen to thirty minutes before being "neutralized." Ammonium thioglycolate is the most common chemical used for this purpose. In general, the weaker the waving solution and the larger the rollers used, the softer are the resulting waves.

If you bleach your hair and also wish to have it permed, you should have it professionally done to minimize the risk of damage to your hair. In addition, fine, limp, brittle, wiry, or damaged hair is difficult to perm. Permanent waving can be very hard on bleached hair.

HAIR STRAIGHTENING

Hair straightening, like permanent waving, requires the breakage of the strong sulfur bonds within hair. Thioglycolates, the same chemicals used for perming, may be used for hair straightening. In addition, bisulfite- and sodium hydroxide–containing relaxing lotions (hair straighteners) may be used.

Thioglycolates are generally relatively safe for use. Unfortunately, they often do not produce the desired degree of straightening. Bisulfite straighteners, also called "curl relaxers," are generally effective and mild on the hair and scalp. For that reason, they enjoy wide use for home straightening. Sodium hydroxide, which works very rapidly, is an extremely potent caustic agent whose use is limited to professional salons. Scalp irritation and burns have resulted from its improper use; blindness can even result if sodium hydroxide gets into the eyes.

Regardless of which relaxing lotion is used, hair straightening involves several basic steps. First, the relaxing lotion is applied to the hair and allowed to work for between ten and twenty minutes. During that time, the hair is continually combed until it begins to hang straight. At that point, the relaxing lotion is neutralized. The final step consists of placing the hair in giant rollers and drying it.

Before leaving the subject of hair straightening, a word should be said about the use of steam ironing for straightening hair. THIS PRACTICE SHOULD BE TOTALLY AVOIDED. The risk of heat damage to your hair, or even accidental burning of your skin and scalp, make this method unacceptable.

HAIR THINNING
AND HAIR LOSS

There are numerous causes for hair thinning and hair loss. Many hair-loss conditions are temporary; unhappily, some are not. If you are experiencing a hair-loss problem, you should consult with a dermatologist. The following is a general discussion of a few of the more common causes of hair loss.

Thin or Fragile Hair

There are two kinds of hair-thinning problems that are really not hair-thinning problems at all: thin hair and fragile hair. In both cases, hair appears to have thinned out and been lost, although no hair loss has actually occurred.

Many people have naturally very fine (thin) hair. Hair thickness is an inherited trait. Blondes characteristically have fine hair. Occasionally, thinness of hairs is mistaken for hair thinning. Although there is no way to permanently thicken hair, the use of protein conditioners and body builders can be helpful to create the impression of greater thickness.

Fragile hair, which tends to break easily, is another problem that can give the false impression of hair loss. Excessively bleached, permed, or straightened hair tends to be extremely fragile, particularly if exposed to frequent combing, brushing, or blow-drying. People who habitually bite, chew, or twirl their hair can also damage it and cause breakage. Regardless of the cause, should many hairs break, a condition *resembling* hair loss can result. Fortunately, simply stopping the bleaching and perming, refraining from any habitual tugging at your

hair, and using conditioners is often all that is necessary
to allow hair to regrow normally.

Traction Alopecia

Traction means pulling, and *alopecia* means baldness.
Traction alopecia, therefore, means hair loss resulting
from prolonged or excessive tension on the hair roots.
Certain styling practices, such as "cornrowing," braid-
ing, or hair plaiting can lead to traction alopecia. So
can ponytails, pigtails, or too frequent use of very tight
rollers. If these troublesome styling practices are stopped
soon enough, the hair usually regrows normally within
several months. If these practices are continued, however, permanent hair loss can result.

Stress-Induced Hair Loss

Telogen effluvium, or stress-induced hair loss, is an extremely alarming form of hair loss. A number of physical
or emotional stresses have been known to precede this
form of hair loss. These include, among many others,
episodes of prolonged high fever, undergoing major,
or even minor, surgery, crash-dieting, pregnancy, and
loss of a loved one. With stress-induced hair loss, hair
may suddenly begin falling out in batches. Up to 40
percent of scalp hairs may be lost by the time the hair
stops falling out. Fortunately, this condition is usually
temporary. Once the stress is eliminated, hair usually
regrows normally within several months.

Alopecia Areata

Alopecia areata is a common hair-loss condition that
can affect people of any age, particularly young adults.
It seems to run in families in as many as one-fifth of all
cases. Alopecia areata is believed to result from a kind
of "allergy to self," in which the body's germ-fighting
immune system goes awry and begins instead to attack
the roots of the hairs, instead of germs. Roundish, stark,
hairless patches typically appear on the scalp or else-
where on the body.

Alopecia areata can be responsible for mild or

extensive hair loss. When the entire scalp is involved, the process is called *alopecia totalis*. When hair is lost over the entire body, the condition is referred to as *alopecia universalis*.

Spontaneous complete recovery occurs in approximately one-third of all patients with alopecia areata. Partial recovery is seen in another third. Unfortunately, repeat attacks are common. Dermatologists have available a number of topical therapies that have been found to be effective in many cases of persistent alopecia areata. Injections of anti-inflammatory corticosteroids in the hairless patches are particularly effective for stimulating regrowth. Oral medications are occasionally needed in more severe cases.

If you are interested in learning more about alopecia areata, you can contact the National Alopecia Areata Foundation at P.O. Box 5027, Mill Valley, California 94941. Local chapters are located all over the United States. At meetings, individuals suffering from alopecia areata obtain the most up-to-date information about developments in research and therapy, draw mutual support, and basically learn to cope with their condition.

LICE

Once believed to be a disease of lower socioeconomic groups and crowding, lice infestation is now known to affect people of all ages, races, and socioeconomic groups. There are three types of lice that naturally infest humans: head lice, body lice, and pubic or "crab" lice. All three types feed by biting the skin and sucking blood. Lice infestation, or *pediculosis,* as doctors call it, is highly catching; all forms cause severe itching. Head and body lice are transmitted from one individual to the next by direct contact with infested hairs or contact with intimate apparel, combs, hats, etc. Pubic lice are spread largely by sexual contact.

Lice reproduce very rapidly, and lice eggs, called nits, hatch every seven to ten days. Mature lice survive for about one month. Body lice deposit their eggs within

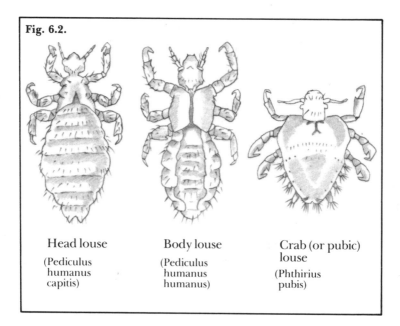

Fig. 6.2.

Head louse	Body louse	Crab (or pubic) louse
(Pediculus humanus capitis)	(Pediculus humanus humanus)	(Phthirius pubis)

The Three Types of Human Lice

the seams of clothing. Head and pubic lice lay their eggs on the hairs within the infested areas.

If you look closely at areas infested by head or pubic lice, you may occasionally see an adult louse, but more often you will find very small, whitish, dandrufflike eggs (the nits) firmly attached to the hair shafts. On the other hand, long scratch marks are the hallmark of body lice infestation. Pubic lice can also infest the eyelashes, armpit, and mustache areas.

Breaks in the skin due to scratching can result in bacterial infections and abscesses. Furthermore, body lice can be carriers of other, more serious, epidemic diseases. These include typhus and relapsing fever. Fortunately, body lice are uncommon in the United States, and pubic and head lice have not been found to be carriers of other diseases.

Naturally, attention to personal cleanliness and

avoidance of direct contact with infected individuals are the best ways to prevent lice infestation. Not sharing intimate apparel, sleepwear, linens, towels, combs, brushes, and other personal items is another effective method.

Two types of medications have proven effective in curing lice infestation. One contains lindane **(Kwell, Scabene),** the same medication recommended for scabies. The second contains pyrethrin **(R D),** another effective pesticide. Although treatment with these agents kills them, the nits often remain attached to the hair shafts. This should be no reason for concern. To dislodge dead nits, you can rinse your hair with a solution containing one part water and one part plain white vinegar, following which you should comb your hair thoroughly with a fine-tooth comb. As with scabies, all intimate apparel and items that came into contact with infested body areas should be hot-water laundered or dry-cleaned.

7

Nail Care

For thousands of years, long, attractive fingernails have been considered signs of not only beauty but of wealth and social position. In fact, nail coloring has been practiced since ancient times. Today, the presence of long, neatly manicured and polished nails remains a symbol of the good life. Well-groomed nails reflect not only a healthy concern for yourself but also a sense of self-confidence.

Not merely ornamental, however, nails serve several useful functions. For one thing, their presence adds to our sense of touch. They also protect the fingertips and, of course, are useful for picking things up. Just as your skin and hair need proper care to remain healthy, so do your nails.

WHAT'S IN A NAIL

Figure 7.1 shows top and side views of a normal fingernail. The *nail plate*, or more simply, the nail, is largely made up of layers of keratin, the same tough protein composing your skin and hair. Like the upper-most layer of your skin and your hair, nails are com-

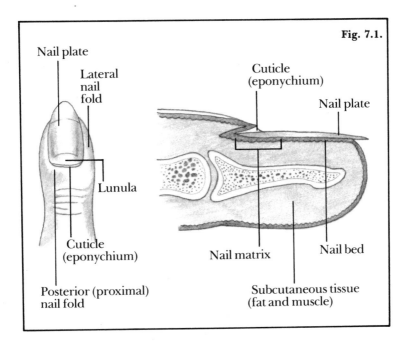

The Human Fingernail

posed of layers of *nonliving* material. Small amounts of calcium, phosphorus, and trace metals such as chromium, selenium, and zinc are also found in the nail plate.

The *nail matrix* is the living and growing area of the nail. There, special cells continuously produce new nail. Any damage to the matrix can result in distorted nail growth and deformed nails. Most of the nail matrix is hidden from view below the skin of the so-called *posterior nail fold*, which is located at the base of the nail plate. The *lunula*, which is the white, crescent-shaped area at the base of the nail plate, is the only area of nail matrix visible to the naked eye. The *cuticle*, the opaque skin fold found at the base of the nail plate, serves to protect the base of the nail from irritation and infection.

The *nail bed* lies directly below the nail plate. It is

soft and grooved and serves to cushion the nail plate. It also contains many small blood vessels that oxygenate and nourish the nail matrix. Following loss of a nail for any reason, the nail bed can harden and form a tough, protective barrier that can compensate for the lost nail.

SOME INTERESTING FACTS
ABOUT NAILS

Nails grow only about ¼ inch (6 mm) each month. The average time for fingernails to grow from the base to the free edge takes about six months. (Toenails take about twelve to eighteen months.) Nails grow faster in hot weather and during childhood and pregnancy. Playing the piano, typing, and nail biting also speed up nail growth. Interestingly, for most of us, the middle fingernail grows the fastest, and, if you are right-handed, the fingernails of your right hand will grow faster than those of your left.

On the other hand, cold weather, general illness, and advancing age slow nail growth. In fact, the rate of nail growth gradually falls by nearly 50 percent between the ages of twenty-five and ninety-five. In general, nails also tend to become thicker, more irregular, and mis-shapen as you get older.

PROPER NAIL CARE

If you want to ensure strong and attractive nails, you must always be mindful of the first and most important rule of good nail care: *Be kind to your nails.* That means making a special effort to protect them and avoid injuring them. It means wearing protective gloves, such as rubber gloves, when performing chores around the house, gardening, or doing hobby work. It means using protective gloves when washing dishes. Exposure to household detergents and solvents can be quite damaging to nails, weakening and roughening them. It means using a pencil to dial the telephone and remembering to pick things up with your fingerpads instead of with your fingernails.

Finally, proper nail care means knowing about the safety and correct use of the various kinds of nail cosmetics. Used incorrectly, they can be the cause of a wide gamut of nail problems.

Clipping, Filing, and Trimming

Clipping your nails, filing them, and trimming the cuticle must be *gently and properly* performed to prevent nail problems. To prevent ingrown nail problems (the embedding of nails into the surrounding flesh), your nails should be clipped or cut straight across, rounding them only slightly at the edges. When filing your nails, use only the fine side of the emery board or a diamond file. Nails should be filed toward the center to round the edges, not toward their edges. Beveling the edges of your nails is best accomplished by passing the fine side of the emery board, held at about a 45° angle, around the nail edges.

Cuticles are especially important protective structures and must be treated delicately. Wide or unsightly cuticles should be pushed back gently to prevent unnecessary pressure and damage to the underlying nail matrix. To soften your cuticles, soak them in warm water for a few minutes. They can then be more easily pushed back with either your fingertips or with a towel; they can also be more easily trimmed when softened.

Nail Strengthening

Your nails may be strengthened by a simple regimen that consists of first soaking them in lukewarm water each night, followed by applying a special moisturizing lotion immediately after, such as **Lac-Hydrin** or **Complex-15,** while the nails are still moist. The use of ordinary moisturizers after soaking, such as **Moisturel** or even plain olive oil, can also be helpful for this purpose. Special cuticle creams and oils intended to soften cuticles and keep them soft are no more effective than regular skin moisturizers. In fact, Moisturel applied to the cuticle serves just as well. In general, special nail creams having a granulated consistency for smoothing nails are seldom necessary.

Of Doubtful Value

For many years gelatin has been recommended for strengthening weakened nails. Sold in powder or capsule forms, gelatin, a protein, is supposed to nourish and harden nails if taken daily. Unfortunately, gelatin remains of unproven value and is probably useless. Furthermore, other supposedly healthful supplements, such as vitamin A and seaweed, have also proven useless. The application of white iodine or hydrogen peroxide to the nails, which was done in the past, is equally useless.

Your nails, as mentioned earlier, contain small amounts of the mineral calcium. Recently, certain individuals have advocated the use of calcium supplements to promote nail growth and hardness. The idea gained some support following the observation that certain women taking calcium supplements for a bone-thinning disease called osteoporosis had noticed faster-growing and stronger nails. The final verdict on the value of calcium supplements for helping nails is not yet in, although most investigators believe that its benefits are probably minimal at best. On the other hand, overconsumption of calcium supplements in a vain attempt to help strengthen nails can be dangerous to your general health and should be avoided unless prescribed by your physician.

NAIL COSMETICS

Nail Polishes

Each year, Americans spend about $200 million for nail polishes, and this figure is expected to continue to climb. In general, nail polishes, or nail enamels as they are also called, add color to your nails and protect them.

The active ingredients in nail polish include nitrocellulose, pigments, resins, and plasticizers. To permit better adherence of the polish to the nail, nail polishes do *not* contain oil/wax moisturizing bases.

Derived from plant cellulose, nitrocellulose is the main film-forming ingredient in nail polish and is waterproof. Nitrocellulose imparts toughness and durability to polish. Resins improve its adhesion and gloss. Plasticizers add gloss and make polish less brittle when it dries. Pigments (colors) and pearlizers (shimmer producers) are added to give nail polish its final color and shade. Finally, some nail polishes also contain nylon fibers for thickening and strenghtening nails.

Nail polishes must be applied evenly to the nail plate. Care should be taken to avoid applying it to the cuticles. If a chip should occur in the finish, it is better just to touch it up than to remove the entire layer of finish with nail polish remover and reapply an all new coat of polish. Overuse of nail polish removers is damaging to the nail and can result in fragile, splitting nails. One final warning: overuse of very darkly colored nail polishes may cause deep discoloration of your natural nails.

Nail polishes occasionally cause allergic reactions. Naturally, if you already know that you are allergic to nail polishes, you should avoid using them altogether. Instead, you can use a buffing paste and chamois buffer to give your nails a high gloss. However, buffing should be performed gently, to prevent irritation.

Nail Polish Removers

Nail polish removers, true to their name, are liquids used to remove dried nail polish. They usually contain acetone or acetone derivatives. Since nail polish removers can be irritating to the skin surrounding your nails as well as to the rest of your hands, you should rinse them off thoroughly after use. Too frequent use of nail polish removers can also damage the nail plate by removing some of the cementing substances that hold the nail plate together. When selecting a nail polish remover, you should look for one that contains an oil or lubricant. These added ingredients help to lessen acetone's drying action.

Base Coats and Top Coats

Base coats are essentially clear nail polishes that are meant to be applied *before* regular nail polish is applied. By coating the nail, base coats help nail polishes adhere better. They also help prevent chipping of both polish and nails.

Top coats differ little from base coats. They are applied directly *over* regular nail polish. Top coats serve to increase the glossiness of the polish and preserve polish finish longer. Unfortunately, base coats and top coats can be irritating and allergenic.

Nail Hardeners

Nail hardeners are liquids containing formaldehyde or formaldehyde-releasing ingredients. Nail hardeners are supposed to prevent nail chipping, fraying, and peeling. When applied to the nail plate, these liquids unquestionably harden nails.

Unfortunately, formaldehyde and its derivatives are common irritants and allergic sensitizers. They can cause a variety of nail problems, including excessive dryness and brittleness, discoloration, discomfort, nail separation from the nail bed, nail loss, and even bleeding under the nail plate. Irritation of the surrounding skin and cuticle and surrounding finger may also occur. Unhappily, these untoward reactions may last for weeks or even months. In order to minimize their potential for irritation, nail hardeners should be avoided altogether or used only occasionally. If you use them, take care to apply them *only* to the nail tips rather than to the entire nail. Finally, avoid getting them on your cuticles or the surrounding skin.

Nail builders are protein-containing liquids that are often advertised as being able to nourish or feed your nails. As mentioned earlier, since nails are composed of nonliving protein, they cannot be "nourished" or "fed." However, the protein in nail builders can serve to fill any shallow pits or other fine surface irregularities present on the nail plate. This allows nail polish to go on more smoothly and adhere better.

Nail Menders

Nail-patch kits or nail menders are used to temporarily repair split or partially torn nails. These kits contain a thick, clear nail polish, special tissue paper, and an applicator stick. The polish, which is first applied above the tear and then to the underside of the nail, acts both as a hardener and adhesive. Following this, special tissue paper is applied to the nail and trimmed. Next, one more coat of the polish is applied over the tissued nail surface. Finally, regular nail polish is applied, as usual, to give the finished effect. If you are careful with the patched nail, it may remain in place for several days. Nail patches are easily removable with nail polish remover.

Artificial Nails

Three basic types of artificial nail products are currently available. One type is a preformed nail. This type of nail must be glued on. A second type is a preformed nail having an adhesive backing. This type can be simply pressed on. The third type is formed on the nail using a mold. Artificial nails are generally composed of water-impermeable plastics.

The prolonged use of artificial nail products can cause injury, even permanent damage, to your natural nails. Because they cover your natural nail and do not permit the evaporation of any natural moisture that accumulates under them, softening and lifting off of the underlying natural nail may occur. Such damage can occur particularly if the artificial nails have been left in place for several days.

Glue-on artificial nail products frequently contain acrylate adhesives. Acrylates can be quite irritating to the underlying nail and to the nearby cuticle and surrounding skin. Allergic reactions to these types of artificial nails are quite common. In fact, they account for the majority of adverse reactions to nail cosmetics in general. The overuse of glue-on nails can result in brittleness, splitting, fraying, and discoloration of the natural nails.

Because no glues are necessary for binding them to the natural nails, the adhesive, or press-on, type of artificial nails generally cause the fewest problems. As a rule, avoid the use of all types of artificial nails. However, if you feel you must use them, use the press-on nails. Nevertheless, these should likewise be removed as soon as possible or within several days. Finally, linen wrapping, which has become so popular lately, may also be irritating in many cases. This practice should also be avoided.

COMMON NAIL PROBLEMS

Nail Injury

Trauma to the nail or nail matrix or repeated exposure to certain chemicals can result in temporary or permanent damage to your nails. Accidents such as striking your fingernail with a hammer or getting it caught in a door often result in bleeding and bruising of the soft tissue under the nail. The often frightening-looking black-and-blue mark that usually forms under the nail following these kinds of injuries may take several weeks or months to disappear. Occasionally, bleeding under the nail continues, causing severe pain from the mounting pressure of the accumulating blood. In this case, your doctor may need to make a small opening through the nail to release the entrapped blood below.

Trauma to the nails can have both immediate and long-term effects on the appearance of the nails themselves. When the matrix has been mildly injured, ridging of the nails, the development of white spots, separation of the nail plate from the nail bed, and even temporary loss of the nail may subsequently develop. These abnormalities may persist for months until a new, healthy nail grows out. Unfortunately, when the matrix has been severely damaged or destroyed by trauma, the regrowth of a normal, healthy nail becomes impossible; the nail remains permanently deformed. The extent of nail deformity depends upon the seriousness of nail matrix damage.

Discolorations

Discolorations of your nails can result from numerous causes. More common conditions occasionally giving rise to nail discolorations include the presence of underlying illnesses, such as certain liver, kidney, or glandular diseases; the ingestion of certain drugs; injury to the nail or matrix; and certain inflammations and infectious diseases, such as fungus infections and psoriasis. Some of these conditions are discussed in the following sections. Fortunately, most of these cases are treatable and should be brought to the attention of a dermatologist.

Interestingly, thin brown streaks running from the base to the tip of the nail are quite common in black people; they are perfectly normal and no cause for concern. These streaks are simply moles ("beauty marks," "birthmarks") under the nails. Similar brown streaks in whites, however, should be brought to the immediate attention of a dermatologist, since they can be a sign of a type of skin cancer.

A few of the more common chemicals and drugs that *occasionally* cause nail discolorations are listed below:

Resorcin (topical antiacne drug)—yellow-brown nails

Tetracycline (common antiacne antibiotic)—yellow-brown nails

Minocycline (antiacne antibiotic)—a bluish-gray discoloration

Beta carotene (vitamin A derivative)—a yellowish discoloration

Nicotine (from cigarettes)—brown nails

Nail polishes, base coats, nail hardeners—yellow-brown nails

Ink—discoloration depends upon the ink color

Brittle and Splitting Nails

Nail brittleness and splitting generally become more of a problem as people age. For younger people, however, contact with harsh detergents or other cleansers and the overuse of nail polish removers, nail hardeners, or artificial nails are common causes of brittleness and splitting. Although there is no cure for brittleness or splitting, the use of protective gloves when appropriate, the routine use of nail polish for nail protection, the infrequent use of nail polish removers, and the avoidance of nail hardeners and artificial nails are advisable. In addition, as mentioned earlier, soaking your nails nightly and liberally applying a moisturizer to them afterward can also be helpful.

Hangnails

Hangnails are splits in the skin along the sides of nails. They are *not* hanging nails, as some people mistakenly assume. In fact, they are not nails at all. Often causing a good deal of discomfort or even pain, hangnails usually form on excessively dry and cracking skin. They may also result from accidental paper cuts, overaggressive manicuring, or the nervous habits of picking and nail biting. Proper nail care as outlined above and the use of protective gloves when washing dishes or clothes help to prevent dryness and hangnail formation.

Treating hangnails is simple. Since the tips of hangnails tend to catch on clothes or other objects, you should *carefully* snip them off. Following clipping, hangnails will usually heal like any other cut. Avoid the temptation to pull the tips off, in order to prevent ripping more deeply into the tender flesh at the base of the hangnail.

Bacterial, Fungal, and Yeast Infections

The nail folds, the skin surrounding your nails, play host to a variety of bacterial, fungal, and yeast infections. If left untreated, these infections usually affect nail appearance, growth, and color. If these organisms attack the nail matrix, permanent nail deformities can occur.

Of course, prevention through proper nail care is the best form of therapy for bacterial or yeast infections. Your doctor may have to drain any accumulated pus and begin oral and topical antibiotic or antiyeast therapies. If treatment is initiated early, the nails gradually regrow normally.

Besides yeasts, other kinds of fungi can directly attack the nail plate. Fungal infections of the nail can produce thickened, lusterless, deformed, ridged, and yellowish nails. In addition, whitish flaking and pitting may be found on the nail surface, and thick, crumbling, powdery debris below it. Fungal infections of the nails are curable in many instances but usually require many months of therapy. Consultation with a dermatologist is important. Treatment often consists of the use of both topical and oral antifungal drugs.

Psoriasis

Psoriasis is an inflammatory condition that can affect the skin, scalp, and nails (see Chapter 5). When it involves the nails, psoriasis can damage the nail plate in a number of ways. In many respects, the damage caused by psoriasis resembles the damage caused by fungal infections.

The more common nail changes seen in psoriasis include pitting, horizontal furrows, crumbling, whitish or yellowish discolorations, and loosening and lifting of nails. In more severe cases, fingernail psoriasis is associated with inflammation of the joints of the fingers. Although no cure is yet available for psoriasis, a variety of therapies have been found to be helpful. Prompt evaluation and treatment by a dermatologist, however, is essential.

8

Foot Care

You stand on them all day. You use them to walk and run. You dance with them. If they feel tired, you feel tired. If they're cold, you're cold. If they hurt, you hurt. Much relied upon but often neglected, your feet serve some extremely important functions. If you're not good to your feet, they won't be good to you. Unfortunately, many people have only the barest notions of how to care for their feet.

GENERAL GUIDELINES FOR CHOOSING HEALTHY FOOTWEAR

Without question, most people choose shoes simply by the way they look. In most cases that means if you like them, you buy them. Although often looked to for their advice about footwear, shoe salespeople are not foot-care physicians; they are out to sell you shoes. The responsibility for choosing the right kinds of footwear falls largely upon you. To help you make healthier footwear choices, you need some basic information about feet and shoes.

Proper Size and Materials

You may not be aware of it, but your feet are not always the same size. The size of your feet can change, depending upon the time of day, your position, and the temperature of the surrounding air. Feet tend to swell somewhat by the end of the day, particularly during hot weather. For that reason, whenever possible, do your shoe shopping toward the end of the day. Interestingly, your feet are not even both the same size to begin with. Since one of your feet is normally a little larger than the other, you should, of course, choose your shoe sizes to fit the larger foot. Finally, your feet are at their widest while you are standing with your full weight upon them. Therefore, you should stand up, not sit, when your feet are being measured.

Here are some additional pointers on proper sizing: Make sure that there is at least one-half inch (1.25 cm) between the end of your longest toe and the front end of the shoe (Fig. 8.1). Your longest toe is not necessarily your big toe; it may be the middle, or less commonly, the third toe. When choosing sandals, your longest toe should not extend beyond the sole of the sandal. Also, make sure that the widest part of your foot (when standing) fits the widest part of the shoe (Fig. 8.2). Your toes should not touch the upper part of the shoe when

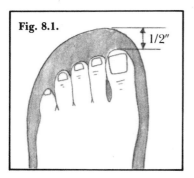

Fig. 8.1.

1/2"

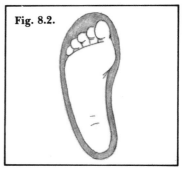

Fig. 8.2.

Proper Shoe Length　　　**Proper Shoe Width**

standing upright. Avoid shoes that taper so sharply toward the front that your toes become crushed together.

After you have been properly measured, you should consider carefully what each shoe is made of and how that might affect you. Ideally, the material composing the upper (the part of the shoe above the sole) should be soft and flexible. Softer, more flexible uppers are generally less irritating to the feet. Unfortunately, not all styles permit the use of soft uppers. In general, suedes, fabrics, crinkle patent leather, and snakeskin are softer and more flexible materials. Less flexible materials include heavy leather, plastics, synthetics, patent leather, and cordovan. Finally, always check the condition of the materials on the inside of the shoes. Make certain that there are no loose linings, wrinkles, protruding stitches, or other irregularities that may rub against or otherwise irritate your feet.

Next, examine the heels and soles of the shoes. Heels and soles are important parts of footwear. They should be constructed for safety and comfort. Leather soles are generally more porous than synthetic soles—that is, they permit more evaporation of sweat. Although less porous, rubber and ripple soles are extremely flexible and comfortable. However, if your feet tend to perspire heavily or if you have a foot odor problem, you should avoid these types of materials. Finally, rubber heel lifts are preferable to leather. They absorb the impact of walking better and they are less likely to cause you to slip on smooth or slick surfaces. Synthetic lifts last longer, but they are less flexible and are particularly unsafe on smooth surfaces.

Because they are generally easier on the feet, three types of footwear deserve special note: loafers, sneakers, and sandals. Properly fitting loafers are fine for normal feet. Owing to their flexibility, so are sneakers. Sandals are also OK, as long as their openings and straps cause no pressure or irritation. However, although sandals do give your feet greater freedom, they provide little protection from trauma.

High heels for everyday use are ill-advised and unhealthy. However, their occasional use as dress-up wear is OK. Daily wearing can lead to permanent foot and back problems because of the way they throw your feet and body forward. People who have worn high heels everyday for many years, even after their feet have become strained from doing so, find it extremely difficult and even painful to return to wearing low heels or flats. This is because after years of walking in high heels, the gait becomes permanently thrust forward to accommodate the high heels; in response, the muscle tendons in the calves of your legs permanently shorten.

If you follow the simple guidelines outlined above for sizing your feet and choosing healthy footwear, you will be less likely to have to "break in" new shoes after you buy them. Breaking in shoes is really another way of saying breaking in your feet. Naturally, if you have any specific questions, or if you have special problems with your feet, you should consult a podiatrist or orthopedic specialist.

Socks and Hosiery

When purchasing socks and hosiery, be aware that nylon hosiery may fit best but does not absorb perspiration. In fact, nylon hosiery can worsen perspiration and odor problems. Cotton, wool, and lisle socks, on the other hand, are more sweat absorbent. If you use these materials, do not tuck any excess or stretched material under your toes; normal flexing of your toes may be hampered in this way.

COMMON FOOT PROBLEMS

Selecting healthy footwear is a very important part of proper foot care. Unfortunately, doing so does not guarantee complete freedom from some common foot problems.

Rough Skin

Dry, scaly skin, particularly on the heels of the feet, is a rather common problem. Sometimes it results from habitually walking barefoot or from wearing loose sandals. Some people seem more prone to rough, scaly skin than others. If you suffer with this problem, you may find that the regular application of a moisturizer to your feet can do much to eliminate it. For best results, moisturizers should be applied immediately after your bath or shower, when the skin is still moist or wet. If the condition persists, see your dermatologist. He or she may prescribe a more potent prescription moisturizer, such as **Lac-hydrin** lotion or a keratolytic agent (a peeling medication) to help remove scales and smooth the roughened skin.

Blisters

Blisters on the feet may be caused by a number of factors. Fungus infections and allergies are occasionally responsible for small blisters. Larger blisters are most commonly due to rubbing and irritation from shoes or boots. These types of blisters are typically quite painful. To minimize the risk of secondary bacterial infection, extreme care must be taken not to tear away the thin blister roof.

To evacuate blister fluid without destroying the blister roof, you should first thoroughly clean the area with alcohol. A new needle may then be used to puncture one or two sides of the blister at its base. Next, the watery blister contents should be gently squeezed out. Finally, the treated area should be recleaned with alcohol, covered with a topical antibiotic, such as **Polysporin** ointment, and protected with a bandage. Blisters treated in this way usually dry up completely in a few days.

Fissures

Fissures are breaks in the skin that occur between the toes or around the heels. They can be extremely painful and can even cause considerable disability. Gait problems or shoe irritation are frequently responsible for heel fissures. Fissures between the toes are usually the result of inadequate drying after bathing or showering.

Conversely, they may also result from overzealous drying with a rough towel. Gently drying the webs between your toes and routinely applying a light dusting of talcum powder usually prevents the formation of fissures.

Depending upon the specific causes of your fissures, your dermatologist or podiatrist may simply advise the use of powders or cornstarch to keep the area dry. The daily application of compound tincture of benzoin may also be recommended. Tincture of benzoin, a sticky liquid, acts as a sealant to protect fissures from further trauma and irritation, permitting faster healing.

Corns and Calluses

Corns and calluses result from persistent and prolonged friction and pressure on the skin of the feet. They frequently form in response to wearing poorly fitted shoes that pinch the two outside toes. In addition, feet that possess any, even subtle, abnormalities in the internal alignments of the bones, ligaments, or tendons are also more prone to developing corns and calluses. This is because such misalignments in the internal anatomy of the feet often lead to abnormal rubbing and irritation within shoes.

When viewed under the microscope, corns and calluses are seen to have the same cellular components. To the naked eye, however, corns appear round or cone-shaped and possess tips (sometimes mistakenly called "roots") that point *into* the skin, instead of outward (Fig. 8.3). These points act like needles or nails driving into the skin. For that reason, corns are frequently extremely painful. Although most corns are found on the outside of the toes, soft corns are found between toes (Fig. 8.4). Soft corns tend to be whitish, moist, soggy, and soft, hence their name. Seed corns—groups of tiny pinhead-size corns—most often develop on the sole (Fig. 8.5).

Calluses are thickenings of skin that form over bony prominences. Calluses are the skin's means of protecting deeper structures from repetitive outside irritation.

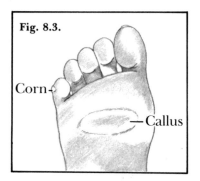

Corns and Calluses

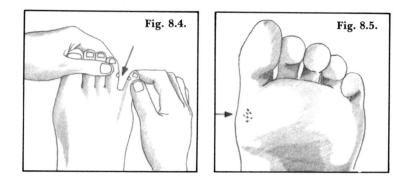

Soft Corns   **Seed Corns**

Calluses are not usually painful, but they can occasionally be extremely so. The heels and center of the balls of the feet (particularly in people who wear high heels) are common locations for callus formation.

Temporary relief from corn and callus discomfort may be obtained by covering them with protective (nonmedicated) corn pads, small circular spot bandages, or moleskin. Soft corns can be temporarily helped by drying the webbed spaces between the toes thoroughly and separating the toe with lamb's wool. Corns and calluses may be softened by first soaking them every night for a ten- or fifteen-minute soak in lukewarm water. While the skin is still moist to wet, corns and calluses may be thinned by gently abrading them with a pumice stone (a piece of volcanic glass pressed into a rough-textured stone; can be purchased in any drugstore) or metal file. Unless advised by your doctor, the use of scissors, razors, callus parers, and medicated pads should be avoided. Naturally, for longer-term relief of corns and calluses, evaluation and treatment by a dermatologist or podiatrist is advised.

Ingrown Toenails

An ingrown toenail forms when the sharp edge of a toenail, most frequently the big toe, penetrates like a knife into the fleshy skin next to it (Fig. 8.6). At first, you may notice slight redness and tenderness. If the condition is allowed to continue, swelling, pain, and a pus-filled discharge will follow. Without proper medical attention, severe infection may result, which could even spread to the underlying bone.

In most cases ingrown toenails are preventable. Ingrown toenails are most commonly caused by tight or ill-fitting shoes. Cutting your nails too short or too far back at their corners is another common cause.

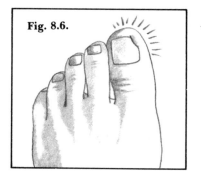

Fig. 8.6.

Ingrown Toenail

Abnormally curved nails, unusually large big toes, and obesity are still other causes of ingrown toenails.

Wearing shoes wide enough and long enough to minimize pressure on your toenails is one very important preventive measure. Cutting your toenails straight across and flush with the underlying pads of the toes, preferably with a nail clipper, is another. The edges of your nail should be left *slightly* rounded, not with sharp points.

Mild cases of ingrown toenails can often be treated at home. Treatment measures include soaking the affected toe daily in warm water. Soaking by itself can be quite soothing. Packing a sterile piece of cotton under the affected nail edge can in some cases lift it away from the surrounding flesh enough to allow for healing and subsequent normal nail growth.

If secondary infection should occur, or if the condition otherwise worsens, see your doctor. Occasionally, the entire nail, or a portion of it, will need to be removed by the doctor, in order to allow it to grow back normally. If you continue to suffer from recurring ingrown toenails, your doctor may suggest the use of caustic chemicals or surgery to permanently remove that portion of the nail that continues to cause you problems.

Two other very common foot conditions, athlete's foot and plantar warts, have already been discussed, in Chapter 5. The management of excessive perspiration, another fairly common foot condition, is covered in Chapter 9.

9

Skin Areas Needing Special Care

It may come as a bit of a surprise to some of you, but your skin is not really one uniform organ from the top of your head to the tip of your toes. Different areas of your skin may differ in a number of ways—in their individual thicknesses, in the number and types of glands they contain, in the amount of hair present, and in the amount of daily wear and tear they undergo. As a result, certain areas of your skin need special attention and care in order to keep them healthy.

MOUTH

Some of you may be questioning why the mouth has been included in a book devoted to skin care. The answer is that the field of dermatology covers not only skin but hair, nails, and all visible mucous membranes. Mucous membranes are moist, membrane-covered, mucus-secreting, skinlike areas. The inside of the mouth, the vagina, and the anus are all mucous membrane regions.

Few people will disagree that a beautiful smile, clean teeth, and fresh breath are important aspects of a person's appearance. Mouth problems that can detract from your appearance, such as cavities, gum disease, bad breath, and loss of teeth, can be minimized or avoided by proper attention to oral hygiene. Some of you may believe that it is the dentist's job to keep your mouth healthy. In reality, the major responsibility for maintaining a healthy mouth lies in *your* hands, not those of your dentist.

Brushing

The aim of good oral hygiene is to remove plaque and prevent its buildup through regular brushing and flossing. Plaque is a thick, tenacious mixture of bacteria, acids, and sugars that adheres to the surface of the teeth; tartar is simply hardened plaque. If not removed, plaque and tartar can lead to the development of bad breath, cavities, gum disease, and (later in life) loss of teeth.

Daily brushing is essential for good oral health. Overall, the regular use of a toothbrush to mechanically clean your teeth and stimulate gums is more important than which toothpaste you use. Moreover, despite the dogma about brushing "after each meal and at bedtime," brushing for four or five minutes once daily, if done properly, is ordinarily sufficient to maintain proper dental health. Some dentists also believe that gently brushing your tongue may help reduce bad breath. If you do not ordinarily brush more than once daily, you should make an effort to rinse your mouth vigorously with water after each meal.

For most people, soft nylon toothbrushes are preferable to stiffer, more abrasive brushes. Furthermore, electric toothbrushes generally offer no particular advantages over manual toothbrushes. In fact, for those who wear braces, the bristles of the electric toothbrush tend to get caught in the braces. On the other hand, electric water-jet devices such as **Water-Pik** can be very useful for cleaning them. If you have any specific questions about what you should use, you should, of course, check with your dentist.

At present, the overwhelming weight of scientific evidence points to the effectiveness of the mineral fluoride for preventing tooth decay. For that reason, many communities fluoridate their drinking water supply and dentists routinely provide periodic fluoride treatments for their patients. Fluoride-containing toothpastes provide additional benefit and are also recommended, particularly for use during the childhood and adolescent cavity-prone years. Incidentally, since all toothpastes contain abrasives, they help dislodge plaque deposits. Despite advertising claims, chewing gums, even sugarless gums, *do not* clean teeth nor supplement brushing and should not be substituted for regular brushing.

Dental Flossing

Despite its benefits, regular brushing is not enough. Although brushing removes plaque from the surface of your teeth, it frequently misses accumulations of food particles and plaque between them. To remove plaque deposits and food particles trapped between teeth, dental flossing is necessary. Waxed and unwaxed types of dental floss are available. Many dentists recommend the use of the unwaxed floss. NOTE: toothpicks are not adequate substitutes for dental floss because they cannot get into the really tight spaces between your teeth. Moreover, other "handy" items that are sometimes used to clean teeth, such as paper clips, pins, and wires, can seriously damage teeth and gums.

Proper flossing consists of several steps: First, cut a long strip of floss and wind each end around the middle fingers of both hands. Holding the floss taut, insert it into the spaces between the teeth; trapped particles can then be dislodged by a front and back sawing motion. Sliding the floss up and down along the sides of each tooth several times dislodges plaque accumulations that could not otherwise be reached by regular brushing. When sliding down the sides of the teeth, you should avoid cutting into your gumline. When a used segment of floss becomes frayed or dirty, one turn around your middle finger brings an unused segment of floss into place. After all the spaces between your teeth have been flossed in this manner, rinse out your mouth thoroughly and vigorously with water.

Mouthwashes and Breath Fresheners

To most Americans, fresh breath has become an important part of their "appearance." The fear of having bad breath (*halitosis*) and "offending" others (much of which is due to television and radio mouthwash advertisers) causes so much concern that the sales for mouthwashes and gargles total into the hundreds of millions of dollars annually. Unfortunately, at best, mouthwashes only *temporarily* mask mouth odor and "freshen" breath.

Bad breath has a variety of causes. Tooth decay, gum diseases, canker sores, herpes infections, severe sore throats, sinus conditions, and stomach disorders are among its causes. These conditions frequently require medical attention, and mouthwashes do little to remedy these situations, although some experts maintain that regular use of mouthwashes can supplement toothbrushing and help to reduce plaque. Mouth sprays, drops, and breath mints, like mouthwashes, only provide a temporary masking aroma to your breath. In general, if you choose to use a mouthwash or freshener, select one with little or no alcohol, since alcohol can be quite drying and irritating for some people.

Some interesting facts about bad breath: A bad taste in your mouth does not automatically mean that you have bad breath, nor does a fresh taste in your mouth guarantee fresh breath. Interestingly, the mouth odors of onions, garlic, and perhaps cigarette smoke do not for the most part arise from trapped particles in the mouth but from the various aromatic chemicals in these foods that are absorbed into the system and exhaled through the lungs. This is why the smell from these foods may linger for hours and cannot be removed with even vigorous toothbrushing.

Finally, most people do have bad breath upon awakening (so-called morning mouth). This form of bad breath results from the overnight action of bacteria upon food particles trapped between teeth. The normal cleansing actions of saliva and swallowing, which occur continually while you are awake, are reduced while you are asleep, contributing further to morning mouth odor. Brushing or rinsing your mouth vigorously before bedtime helps somewhat.

GENITAL AREA

Genital Deodorants

Genital deodorants, or feminine hygiene sprays, as they are frequently called, represent another attempt by advertisers to create a market for a type of product that isn't necessary in the first place. Genital deodorants are available as aerosol sprays, aerosol powder sprays, and premoistened towelettes. These products generally contain antiseptics and fragrances.

Most healthy women, to varying degrees, have natural vaginal odors. Vaginal odor comes from the action of skin bacteria that break down the secretions of the special sweat glands located around the vulva (the vagina and its surrounding lips). Tight-fitting jeans, underwear, and panty hose can contribute to an odor problem by reducing sweat evaporation and providing a warm, moist environment for odor-causing bacteria to flourish. Occasionally, besides odor, tight-fitting garments can cause vulval inflammation, itching, or infection ("panty hose dermatitis"). Nevertheless, gentle soap-and-water cleansing is more effective, and certainly safer, for controlling these odors (and preventing infection) than deodorant sprays. Allergies, swelling, irritation, burns, and stinging have all been known to result from the use of vaginal deodorant sprays.

Foul-smelling vaginal odors may also arise from conditions such as vaginal infections and vaginitis. Medical attention should be sought promptly for these conditions. In addition, forgotten tampons or diaphragms, and occasionally menstrual flow, may be responsible for odors. Removal of the foreign object and simple soap-and-water cleansing usually rectify these conditions. The bottom line: Avoid feminine deodorant sprays and seek medical advice if you have any questions.

Vaginal Douching

In general, vaginal douching is unnecessary for routine genital hygiene. Occasionally, gynecologists or dermatologists may prescribe douches to treat certain bacterial or fungal infections of the vagina. However, with routine use, the ingredients contained in commercial douches can sometimes cause irritation. In some cases, they can injure the lining cells of the vagina and even predispose someone to vaginal infections in a number of ways, such as by upsetting the vagina's delicate acid-base balance, by removing its natural lubricants, or by eliminating the normal bacteria that colonize it.

Commercially available douches typically contain five types of ingredients: detergents and alkalis for cleansing, antiseptics for suppressing bacteria, emollients for lubrication, acids for approximating the normal acid environment of the vagina, and fragrance. If you use a douche, do not use it more than once or twice a week unless recommended by your doctor.

Tampons and Toxic Shock Syndrome (TSS)

Toxic shock syndrome (TSS) is a serious medical condition that has gotten considerable press coverage during the past several years because of its association with the use of superabsorbency menstrual tampons. More recently, TSS has also been linked with the use of sponge contraceptives. TSS largely affects women under thirty and is fatal in nearly 10 percent of cases. The major signs of TSS include the sudden appearance of high fever and a rapid drop in blood pressure, leading to shock, vomiting, diarrhea, severe sunburnlike rash, and extensive skin peeling. TSS is caused by a toxin (a poison) secreted by the bacterium *Staphylococcus aureus*.

Although the true relationship of TSS to the use of superabsorbent tampons is still under investigation, a higher incidence of TSS has been found in women using superabsorbency tampons. However, it remains unclear whether any specific brand is more likely than others to be associated with it. Overall, the risk of TSS seems to be increased by the use of tampons throughout the entire menstrual period.

Until more is learned, if you prefer tampons, use them with discretion. Whenever possible, use menstrual pads for your light days and for nighttime use. Should you develop a fever or rash, or experience nausea or vomiting, during your period, discontinue tampon use and contact your doctor immediately.

UNDERARM PROBLEMS

Sweating and odor represent the two most common underarm problems. Like the genital area, the underarms possess special sweat glands, called *apocrine* glands, which become active after puberty. Apocrine sweat by itself is odorless. However, bacterial breakdown of apocrine sweat causes underarm odor. Bacteria are particularly active in the warm, moist areas of the underarms and groin, where evaporation does not readily occur. Deodorant soaps, deodorants, and antiperspirants have been formulated to deal with perspiration and odor.

Deodorant Soaps

Without question, regular soap-and-water cleansing is one of the most effective ways to reduce underarm odor. Clearly, there can be no odor produced when perspiration and bacteria are simply washed away. Of course, both bacteria and perspiration soon return. Deodorant soaps that contain antibacterials such as triclocarbon (**Safeguard** and **Dial**) or triclosan (**Lifebuoy**), may be helpful in suppressing bacteria and prolonging the anti-odor effects of soap-and-water cleansing. Some people, however, may find these soaps too irritating and drying. In general, avoid these soaps if you have naturally dry or sensitive skin.

Deodorants

Simply defined, deodorants are cosmetics that are intended to reduce body odor. Deodorants may contain fragrances for masking odor or antiseptics for reducing the number of odor-producing bacteria. Fewer bacteria mean less sweat broken down by them to cause odor. Triclosan is a common antiseptic found in many deodorants. Underarm deodorants today are seldom exclusively antibacterial deodorants. Most contain antiperspirants as well.

Antiperspirants

As the name implies, antiperspirants are formulated to reduce perspiration wetness. Although various brands of antiperspirants differ in their abilities to control sweating, to be considered a true antiperspirant a product must reduce the amount of sweating by at least 20 percent. No antiperspirant, however, completely eliminates it.

By reducing the amount of sweat produced, antiperspirants ensure that bacteria have less to work on, making odor less likely. Most antiperspirants contain aluminum chlorohydrate or aluminum chloride. Lotions, creams, sticks, and roll-ons generally appear to be more effective antiperspirants than aerosols. Since they pose no inhalation risks, they are probably safer to use as well.

Surprisingly, adding more active ingredients to a particular antiperspirant does not necessarily make that product more effective. In other words, antiperspirants labeled "extra dry" or "extra-extra dry" may not necessarily be better than their less "extra" counterparts. Antiperspirants also generally require several hours and several applications to reach their maximum effectiveness. Thus, to increase your antiperspirant's effectiveness, apply it first at night and then again the following morning.

Excessive Sweating

Some people suffer from excessive sweating, or *hyperhidrosis*. In most cases, the causes of excessive sweating are unknown. For people who suffer from profuse sweating, the problems of persistent wetness, odor, and clothing stains can cause extreme and continued embarrassment. Frequently, individuals with an underarm sweating problem also suffer with profuse sweating of their hands and feet.

If you have hyperhidrosis, your dermatologist may prescribe antiperspirants that are stronger than those commercially available. Some people are helped by the higher concentrations of aluminum chloride found in **Xerac-ac** lotion or **Drysol**. These products are more effective when applied at bedtime and again in the morning for the reasons discussed earlier. Unfortunately, many people find these antiperspirants too irritating, especially when applied to the sensitive armpit area. For more severe cases of sweating, or for those people who have not responded well to topical therapies, the doctor may prescribe certain oral medications.

Iontophoresis, which consists of exposing the excessively sweaty areas of the body to a small electric current, is sometimes successful. The exact mechanism by which iontophoresis works remains unclear but may have something to do with inducing a temporary clogging of the sweat glands. Until recently, iontophoresis could only be performed in the dermatologist's office or hospital.

In the past few years, however, **Drionics,** a home iontophoresis device, has become available in the United States for the treatment of excessive sweating. Early reports concerning the success of this product have been encouraging in a number of cases. Unfortunately, iontophoresis is not successful in all patients. It is a treatment, not a cure, for hyperhidrosis. Even when successful, treatments must be repeated every four to six weeks.

REMOVING UNWANTED FACIAL HAIR

For many women, the presence of unwanted or excess facial hair can be one of the most psychologically troubling problems. Usually located on the upper lip, chin, and cheeks, these hairs tend to be coarser and darker than normal hairs. Some populations, such as Mediterraneans, are racially more prone to it. Often there is a family history of excess facial hair production. Hormonal factors may also play a role. Happily, a variety of methods are available for removing unwanted hair.

If you have a facial hair problem, you should see a dermatologist. Certain more serious medical conditions have been associated with the production of unwanted, or excessive, hair growth, and these need to be excluded first before concentrating on the cosmetic problem. Clues to the presence of underlying problems include a sudden increase in the amount, coarseness, or distribution of body hair, the sudden appearance of unwanted hair and severe acne, the onset of irregular periods, or a deepening of the voice. Naturally, once any underlying medical conditions have been excluded, attention may be safely turned to the various methods for hair removal.

Mechanical Methods of Hair Removal

Pumicing and Tweezing. Pumicing and tweezing are two inexpensive, mechanical ways of temporarily removing unwanted hair. Pumice stones, made from volcanic rock, are abrasive materials that can be used to rub and wear away fine (less coarse) unwanted hairs. Hairs removed in this way regrow, and pumicing must be repeated every few days. Pumicing is also time-consuming and can be irritating to the skin. A rich moisturizing cream or lotion should be used afterward to lessen irritation.

Tweezing or plucking is an old, but extremely cheap, quick, and effective means for temporary hair removal. Occasionally, repeated tweezing of the same hairs can damage the hair root so much that hair loss at those sites may be permanent. In most cases, however, tweezing needs to be repeated every six to eight weeks. Unfortunately, tweezing and pumicing tend to be very uncomfortable and sometimes even very painful. As a result, only a few hairs can usually be done at one time. In addition, pimples, pustules, and ingrown hairs often form at tweezed sites.

Waxing. Although occasionally performed at home, most waxing is performed in professional salons and is expensive. Waxing consists of applying a hot, melted wax to the site of the unwanted hairs. As the wax cools and hardens, hairs become embedded within it. Once cooled, the wax is pulled away from the skin, carrying along the embedded hairs down to their roots. The skin is left quite smooth. Cold waxing actually differs little from hot waxing except for the addition of an adhesive strip to the wax application. In general, waxing must usually be repeated every six weeks.

Waxing has several drawbacks. For one, it may be painful and irritating to the skin. For another, before waxing, the unwanted hairs must be allowed to grow to an unsightly length of approximately ¼ inch (6mm) to ½ inch (1.25cm) above the skin surface so that they have sufficient length to become adequately embedded within the wax. This often causes embarrassment.

Shaving. Shaving is the fastest, easiest, and one of the cheapest methods of removing hair from large areas. It has the added advantage of being painless. To prevent stubble from becoming obvious, shaving must be repeated every one to two days. Unfortunately, many women with excess facial hair dislike the masculine connotation of shaving. However, contrary to popular belief, once an area is shaved, hairs *do not* regrow faster or thicker thereafter.

For shaving, the choice of electric razor or safety razor is largely one of personal preference. Electric razors are generally less irritating to the skin and less likely to result in nicks and cuts. On the other hand, they usually don't give as smooth a shave as safety razors. Before using a safety razor, your skin should be thoroughly moistened with water and richly lathered with shaving cream. By contrast, if you choose an electric razor, your skin should be completely dry before shaving.

Chemical Methods of Dealing with Unwanted Hair

Bleaching. Although bleaching is not a means of removing hair, it is a simple and common means of dealing with unwanted facial hair. Bleaching is cheap, easy to perform, and creates no stubble or roughness. In general, the less striking the contrast between the bleached hairs and your normal skin color, the more satisfying the cosmetic result. Thus, bleaching usually works best if you have a light complexion. The effects of bleaching generally last between one and four weeks.

On the downside, bleaching is time-consuming, and if the bleach is not left on long enough, hairs become reddish in color rather than blonde. Also, a number of people are sensitive or develop sensitivities to the peroxide and ammonia ingredients contained in home or commercial bleaches. To minimize skin irritation, you should always apply a good moisturizer after bleaching. Before bleaching a large area of skin, you should apply a small amount of bleach to a tiny test area of skin. If no irritation results after about thirty minutes of contact with your skin, you may proceed to bleach the entire desired area.

Chemical Depilatories (Hair Removers). Available in cream, lotion, and foam formulas, chemical hair removers are inexpensive and simple to use. They remove unwanted hairs by reducing them to a jellylike mass that can be easily wiped away. Since they work above and below the surface, they leave your skin smooth, although usually not quite as smooth as after waxing. Like bleaches, however, they have the potential for irritating the skin; a test application before first using them is advisable. In addition, a good moisturizer should be used afterward to minimize irritation.

Electrolysis is the only currently available, proven means of *permanent* hair removal; this remains its primary advantage. Electrolysis consists of sliding a small electric needle down the hair follicle and destroying the hair root with an electric current. In general, an experienced electrologist may be able to treat several hundred hairs in one session. A session usually lasts about forty-five minutes.

Unfortunately, professional electrolysis tends to be expensive, often painful, and requires many treatment sessions. In many cases of extensive facial hair, a year or more of frequent, periodic treatments may be required. Regrowth of hairs occurs approximately 40 percent of the time. Pimples, ingrown hairs, and even scarring are occasional complications of electrolysis.

For women with fewer unwanted hairs, home electrolysis units are available. These units generally work slowly and require patience; only about fifty hairs can be done per hour. **Permatweez,** a battery-powered unit, claims to have a self-correcting, protective spring-action mechanism. According to the manufacturer, this design allows the rounded needle to spring right down to the hair root *only* when the needle has been *properly* inserted into the opening of the pore. After only a few practice sessions, most people can become quite proficient at using these devices.

Finally, a relatively new method of hair removal, using radiofrequency waves, is now available for home use. Radio waves instead of an electric current are transmitted down to the hair roots through a specially designed tweezer. The manufacturer of one such product claims that their device is safe, effective, easy to use, and free of the drawbacks of electrolysis. According to the manufacturer, hairs treated by this method tend to grow back less coarse, and do not regrow at all after repeated treatments. Whether this method of hair removal will live up to its manufacturer's claims remains to be seen.

10

Common Cosmetic Surgical Procedures

Each year, more than 1.5 million Americans have cosmetic surgery performed to change the way they look. Cosmetic surgery, or "plastic" surgery as it was more commonly called in the past, covers a wide variety of medical and surgical procedures to change your appearance. Some of these procedures consist of nothing more than a simple injection; others involve complicated or delicate surgery and require days to weeks of recuperation. Some of the more common cosmetic procedures are discussed in this chapter. These include a variety of surgical treatments for acne scarring, methods of removing moles and other unwanted growths, "nose jobs," chin enlargement or reduction, "ear pinning," and treating port-wine stains.

KNOW THYSELF

Socrates, the famous Greek philosopher and teacher, espoused the concept of "Know thyself," meaning that people should make an effort to understand their own motives and actions, or, what makes them tick. The meaning of that phrase is particularly important to reflect upon before undergoing cosmetic surgery. You will almost surely experience dissatisfaction or disappointment with the results of any cosmetic surgery if you are unsure about whether you really wanted a particular procedure done in the first place or if you weren't quite ready for it. Disappointment also lurks close by if you mistake a cosmetic surgeon for a miracle worker, capable of turning a plain person into a stunning movie star. Disappointment will also likely follow if you believe that changing your appearance will automatically or necessarily win you more friends or dates, etc. In short, to prevent dissatisfaction and disappointment, be sure of what *you* (not your friends or relatives) really want and be realistic about the results if you decide to have cosmetic surgery.

CHOOSING THE RIGHT DOCTOR

No single physician is right for everyone. Sometimes you must do quite a bit of searching to find the best one for your needs. Even if you are careful about choosing, however, finding the right cosmetic surgeon can be quite confusing these days. For one thing, in the past, plastic surgeons dominated the field of cosmetic surgery. So if you wanted any kind of cosmetic work done, you simply went to a plastic surgeon. Today, things are different. Many fields of medicine have subspecialties that are devoted to cosmetic surgery. For example, many training programs in otolaryngology (ear, nose, and throat), ophthalmology (eye), oral surgery (advanced dental surgery), and dermatology regularly include sessions on cosmetic surgery. Thus today, for example, if you want a "nose job," you might consult with a plastic surgeon or an otolaryngologist; for chin surgery, you could consult with a plastic surgeon, otolaryngologist, or oral surgeon.

Although, in general, the well-trained and experienced surgeon in any of these specialties is technically capable of performing the desired procedure, some suggestions for selecting a cosmetic surgeon are in order. Probably the best way to choose a surgeon is to see some of his or her work. If you have any friends or relatives who have had cosmetic surgery, ask them whether they were satisfied with the care they received and the results. Or you might ask a trusted family physician for a recommendation. Family physicians and internists frequently know the reputations, if not the work, of several local cosmetic surgeons. Finally, as a last resort, you can contact your local county medical society and ask for a board-certified, university-affiliated physician who performs the kind of surgery you wish to have.

A word to the wise. There has been a recent upsurge of heavy TV, radio, and print media advertising for some cosmetic surgery clinics with offices all over the country. Many of these places offer free consultations, quick appointments, same-day service, free limousine pickup, and bargain fees. But beware. Don't trust any place that guarantees results or downplays the risks. Don't let yourself be talked into any cosmetic procedure you don't really want or think you need. Furthermore, check their fees; they may not be such bargains after all.

COSMETIC SURGERY FOR ACNE SCARS

Collagen Injections

Several years ago and after six years of extensive testing, the FDA approved the use of injectable **Zyderm** collagen implants for the treatment of wrinkles and scars. Injectable collagen has been successfully used to plump up depressed acne scars (pockmarks) and make them less noticeable.

The collagen used in Zyderm is a highly purified form of collagen derived from calfskin. Collagen is a natural structural protein making up cartilage, bone, and fibrous tissue. Zyderm collagen injections are used to supplement the body's natural collagen. At present, more than 300,000 people have received collagen implant injections. More recently, an additional product, **Zyplast,** was approved by the FDA for use in deeper wrinkles, depressions, and scars. After taking a careful history about your general health, your doctor will administer a small test amount in your forearm to make sure that you do not have any allergies to any of the components in the material. One month later, if no allergy is discovered, actual treatment on the face can begin.

Not to be confused with the collagen contained in some moisturizers, which is meant to be applied to the surface of the skin (and *cannot* be absorbed by it), the collagen in Zyderm is injected *under* the skin, precisely where it is needed. A small mosquito bite–like bump forms at the site of the injection, which settles down between twenty-four and seventy-two hours after injection. Because they are tightly bound to the underlying skin, acne scars often require more than one treatment; the first treatment softens the scar, the second or third plumps it up to the desired level. Treatment sessions are usually spaced at two- to four-week intervals.

The cosmetic benefit of collagen injections is temporary. Effects may last for months to years before retreatment is necessary, depending, of course, on your individual circumstances. Unfortunately, deep, "ice-pick" scars do not respond well to collagen injections; their treatment is discussed later.

Zyderm collagen injections should not be confused with silicone injections, which have long been used for many of the same purposes. However, after nearly thirty years of use, silicone injections have still not been granted approval by the FDA for use in treating wrinkles or acne scars. Unlike collagen, which is a natural and biodegradable material, silicone is not biodegradable. Once injected into the skin it remains there permanently and cannot be removed. It has also been known to shift, causing odd-appearing bumps in the skin at sites distant from the original injection sites. For these reasons, it is not recommended here.

Dermabrasion
Dermabrasion is a form of skin sanding used to smooth irregular or pockmarked skin. Those with fair skin and

shallower pock scars are generally considered the best candidates for dermabrasion. More darkly complected individuals have a greater risk of developing dark patches on their skin after dermabrasion, although this occurs only occasionally.

Depressed acne scars are generally highly visible because when light strikes them from the side, prominent shadows are formed within the scars, making them stand out more. Dermabrasion, which is accomplished by the use of wire brushes and diamond-headed cutting wheels, serves to smooth and grade the edges of the scar craters so that they appear less prominent when lit from the side.

Crusts develop sometime within the first week after dermabrasion and are shed by the end of the third week. If performed on a Thursday, most students can return to school by the following Monday. To prevent the formation of blotchy skin discolorations, sun exposure must be avoided for approximately three months after dermabrasion.

Chemical Peels

Very shallow types of acne scarring may be improved through the use of chemical peels. In a chemical peel, a strong acid, frequently trichloroacetic acid, is applied to the skin either with a cotton-tipped applicator or a brush. The irritation that follows is equivalent to a strong burn. After chemical peel, treated skin flakes off during the next one to two weeks. The new underlying skin is usually smoother and fresher-looking, and very shallow, depressed scars may appear somewhat less prominent. Chemical peels are not effective for deeper scars.

Removing "Ice-Pick" Scars

As mentioned earlier, "ice-pick" scars are deep scars resulting from prior acne damage. They typically have narrow openings. Hence, Zyderm injections, dermabrasions, and chemical peels—procedures that are better suited to improving shallow scars—are generally ineffective for treating ice-pick scars. However, three simple, closely related cosmetic procedures have been shown to produce satisfactory cosmetic results: punch excision, punch elevation, and punch grafting. Each of these procedures takes only a few minutes to perform, and the cosmetic results can be quite gratifying.

A *punch* is a cookie cutter–like surgical instrument used to cut out a small plug of skin. In a punch excision, following the administration of a local anesthetic (similar to the Novocain that the dentist gives you), the pit scar is cut out with the punch, the scar-containing plug is discarded, and the remaining opening is closed with ultrafine sutures (stitches). In a punch elevation, instead of discarding the plug of scar tissue, it is elevated to the surface of the skin and fixed in place either with special tape or regular stitches. Several weeks later the elevated plug is finely sanded flush with the surrounding skin.

In punch grafting, a plug of skin is once again removed with a punch and discarded, but this time the resulting opening is filled with a plug of new skin (called a *graft*) taken from behind the ear. Skin from behind the ear matches facial skin quite closely. Until healing has taken place, the graft is either stitched or taped in place.

Keloids and "Proud Flesh"

Although it usually produces depressed scars, severe, uncontrolled acne can also lead to the development of two kinds of raised scars: keloids and hypertrophic scars ("proud flesh"). Very firm and pink in color, hypertrophic scars represent a complication of wound healing in which healing skin overshoots its mark and produces excess healing tissue that protrudes above the skin surface, hence the name "proud" flesh. Usually after many months, proud flesh spontaneously sinks back to a level flush with the surrounding normal skin. If this does not occur, however, the dermatologist can inject a small amount of an anti-inflammatory corticosteroid solution, which causes the proud flesh scar to shrink.

Keloids are very firm, flesh- to ivory-colored scars

that can become quite disfiguring. The tendency to form keloids appears to have a racial and genetic predisposition. Keloids more commonly occur in blacks and Asians, although whites are by no means exempt.

Whereas hypertrophic scars tend to remain confined to the location of the prior acne damage, keloids often extend well beyond the confines of the original acne damage. Like hypertrophic scars, keloids may be shrunk through the injection of corticosteroid solutions. As a rule, keloids do not shrink by themselves.

"NOSE JOBS"

The nose and the chin are considered the two main "character" features of the face. A nose job, or *rhinoplasty,* as cosmetic surgeons call it, is used to correct nasal deformities, either for medical or purely cosmetic concerns. Noses that are too wide, thick, long, bumpy, or hooked are among the types that can be improved by rhinoplasty (Fig. 10.1). Nose jobs basically consist of removing excess nasal bone and cartilage, rearranging the nose, and reshaping it.

Nose jobs are usually performed under local anesthesia, although sometimes general anesthesia is used. A typical operation takes between one and three hours to perform. Even though it is considered a minor surgical procedure, rhinoplasty requires two or three days of hospitalization. After the surgery, patients experience a considerable amount of swelling and bruising of the nose, cheeks, and eyelids.

All wound dressings are removed by the end of the first week, and most students can return to school within two to three weeks after the operation. Contact sports must be avoided, however, for about three months. The nose assumes its final appearance by about six months, when most of the swelling has disappeared.

COSMETIC CHIN SURGERY

There are basically two types of cosmetic surgery to improve chin appearance: procedures to reduce chin

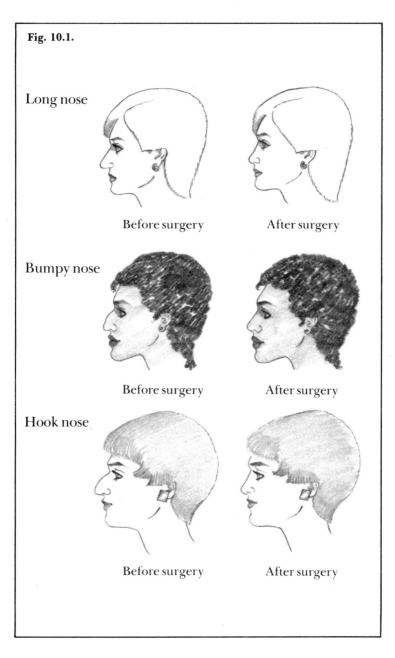

Fig. 10.1.

Long nose

Before surgery   After surgery

Bumpy nose

Before surgery   After surgery

Hook nose

Before surgery   After surgery

Examples of "Nose Jobs"

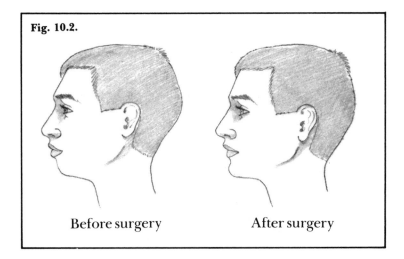

Fig. 10.2.

Before surgery   After surgery

Mentoplasty for Receding Chin

size and procedures to increase it. The medical term *mentoplasty*, or cosmetic chin surgery, refers to both types of procedures.

A "weak" chin, also called a recessive chin, is the single most common chin problem for which people seek cosmetic surgical correction (Fig. 10.2). Interestingly, since the nose and chin are closely interrelated facial features, often the presence of a recessive chin will first become more obvious after a nose job.

Chin augmentation to correct a recessed chin consists of the insertion of a silicone prosthesis into a pocket created in front of the natural chin bone. The silicone prosthesis may be inserted through a small incision made under the chin or through an incision made within the mouth at the point where the base of the lower lip and teeth join. Chin augmentation surgery, ordinarily performed under local anesthesia, usually takes about one to one and a half hours to complete and requires only an overnight hospital stay. Incidentally, the silicone used in mentoplasty differs from, and should not be confused with, the injectable silicone droplets used for treating acne scars. Silicone prostheses for chin augmentation are approved by the FDA.

Chin reduction to reduce an elongated, pointy chin ("witch's" chin) or a protruding chin is performed in a similar fashion to chin augmentation. However, instead of inserting a prosthesis, the natural chin is chiseled down to the desired size and shape. The cosmetic results of this chin-reduction surgery are generally quite gratifying.

EAR PINNING

Otoplasty, or "ear pinning," for correcting ear deformities is one of the most common cosmetic surgical procedures performed today. Otoplasty is used to correct protruding, "flyaway," or "Dumbo"-shaped ears.

Otoplasty usually requires between one and three hours to perform. The procedure essentially consists of thinning out and removing excess cartilage from the ear so that the ear can be repositioned closer to the scalp. Following a two- or three-day hospitalization, patients are usually permitted to go home. Students can return to school about five days later. For about two months, however, a nighttime elastic pressure bandage must be worn.

REMOVING MOLES AND MILIA

A mole, or *nevus,* is a benign overgrowth of pigment cells. Most of you are probably more familiar with its other popular names: birthmark and beauty mark. Moles may be flat or raised and vary from flesh-colored to a very dark brown. Depending upon their location, particularly on the face, moles can be quite prominent and unattractive. Fortunately, cosmetic procedures are available so that people do not have to live with unsightly or unwanted moles.

Moles may be removed in the dermatologist's office in a matter of minutes, under local anesthesia. Some cosmetic surgeons elect to cut deeply into the skin to remove the "root" of the mole. This is generally a more involved procedure requiring the placement of stitches. Others merely "sculpt" away the surface of the mole and contour its base to approximate the contours of the surrounding skin. The sculpting technique requires no stitches and takes only about five minutes to perform. The cosmetic results of this method have been excellent.

Milia (sing. *milium*) are small cysts that may be found in individuals of any age. They are generally firm, tiny, round, and whitish raised bumps that contain a kernel of densely packed hair follicle skin cells and protein. Their presence, particularly on the face, is of cosmetic significance only.

Dermatologists can easily remove milia in the office by opening their surfaces with a fine scalpel blade and extruding the contents. Care is taken to remove the entire kernel and its surrounding sac in order to minimize the possibility of recurrence. Depending upon individual circumstances, especially when numerous milia are present, many dermatologists elect to destroy milia by electrodesiccation, that is, by inserting an ultrafine needle into them and applying a mild electric current.

TREATING PORT-WINE STAINS

Nevus flammeus, or port-wine stain, as it is more commonly known, is a birthmark composed of numerous bunched-up, tiny blood vessels. Port-wine stains are the most common type of blood vessel birthmark. Flat or bumpy in texture, red or purplish in color, port-wine stains range in size from a half inch (1.25 cm) to many inches in diameter. Fortunately, they are most often located on the neck or back of the scalp, where they are less noticeable. When they are large and involve the face, however, they can be severely disfiguring and the source of much psychological anguish.

Unhappily, no therapy currently available is capable of completely eliminating or blanching port-wine stains. However, relatively recently, the argon laser has been found to be quite effective for treating certain types of port-wine stains. Lasers are intense, focused beams of light. The argon laser emits a light that is absorbed largely by hemoglobin, the red pigment in red blood cells. Thus, the argon laser light can be aimed just where it is needed, within the abnormal blood vessels. As a result, surrounding tissue is hardly damaged and the possibility of post-treatment scarring is greatly reduced. And by blanching port-wine stains or flattening the more bumpy ones with the argon laser, most people with this problem subsequently find that the application of masking cosmetics becomes easier and more effective. Large port-wine stains may require a year or more of periodic laser treatments, which are usually quite costly.

Index

Cosmetics, 26, 30–43, *40*
  acne and, 38, 39, 55
  astringents, fresheners, and
    toners, 41–42, 55–56, 57
  for nails, 100–04
Cosmetic surgery, 130–41, *138*

Dandruff, 70–71, 72
Deodorants, 123–24
  genital, 121–22
Depilatories, 128
Dermabrasion, 133–34
Dermatitis (eczema), 27, 66–71
Dermis, 13, 15
Detergent soaps, 22
Douching, 122
Drinking, 24, 27–29
Drugs, 24, 29
Dyes, hair, 87–88

Eczema. *See* Dermatitis
Electrolysis, 129
Emollients, 33, 34
Emotions, 9, 26–27
  acne and, 49
  hair loss and, 92
Emulsifying agents, 33, 34–35
Emulsion stabilizers, 33, 35
Epidermis, 13–14
Erythromycin, 62, 63
Exercise, 25–26
Exotic additives, 32–33, 36

Fatty acids, 48, 58
Feet, 108–16, *109*
Fissures, 112–13
Fluoride treatments, 119
Flushing, 27–28
Folliculitis, 77
Foods, acne and, 50–51
Fungal infections, 74–76, 106–07
Furunculosis, 77

Gelatin, 100
Gellants, 35–36
Genetic factors, 46, 70, 72, 91
Genital area, 121–23

Hair, 70–71, 81–95, *82*
  facial, removing, 125–29
  lice in, 93–95, *94*
Hair follicles, 77, 81, *82*

Hair follicles (*continued*)
  acne development in, 46–48,
    58
  prickly (keratosis pilaris), 71–
    72
Halitosis, 120–21
Heredity, 46, 70, 72, 91
Herpes, 17
Horny layer, 13
Humectants, 33, 34, 37
Hyperhidrosis, 124–25
Hypertrophic scars, 135, 136

"Ice-pick" scars, 133, 134–35
Impetigo, 77
Inactive ingredients, 32–33
Incision and drainage procedures,
    65
Infections, 46, 74–80, 106–7
Inflammations, 46
Ingrown toenails, *115*–16
Injections
  in cosmetic surgery, 132–33
  therapeutic, 65
Iodine, 25, 51
Iontophoresis, 125
Irritant contact dermatitis, 69–70
Itching, 27

Jewelry, 26
Jock itch, 74

Keloids, 135–36
Keratosis pilaris, 71–72

Lice, 93–95, *94*
Lunula, 97

Makeup. *See* Cosmetics
Malignant melanoma, 17
Masks, 37–38, 57–58, 59
Melanin, 14
Melanocytes, 13–14
Mentoplasty, 136–39, *138*
Milia, 140
Minerals, 24–25
Minocycline, 62
Moisturizers, 15, 22–24, 33, 37
  acne and, 23, 24, 37, 55
  conditioners as, 86–87
  for nails, 99–100, 106
Moles, 139–40
Mouth care. *See* Oral hygiene